Dermatology

ILLUSTRATED CLINICAL CASES

Dermatology

EDITED BY

WILLIAM W. HUANG MD, MPH
Associate Professor and Residency Program Director
Department of Dermatology
Wake Forest University School of Medicine
Winston-Salem, North Carolina, USA

STEVEN R. FELDMAN MD, PhD
Professor of Dermatology, Pathology, and Public Health Sciences
Wake Forest University School of Medicine
Winston-Salem, North Carolina, USA

CHRISTINE S. AHN MD
Dermatology Resident
Department of Dermatology
Wake Forest University School of Medicine
Winston-Salem, North Carolina, USA

ROBIN S. LEWALLEN MD
Dermatology Resident and Co-Chief Resident
Department of Dermatology
Wake Forest University School of Medicine
Winston-Salem, North Carolina, USA

CRC Press
Taylor & Francis Group
Boca Raton London New York

CRC Press is an imprint of the
Taylor & Francis Group, an **informa** business

CRC Press
Taylor & Francis Group
6000 Broken Sound Parkway NW, Suite 300
Boca Raton, FL 33487-2742

Printed in Great Britain by Ashford Colour Press Ltd
Version Date: 20160826

International Standard Book Number-13: 978-1-4987-2288-9 (Paperback)

Library of Congress Cataloging-in-Publication Data

Names: Huang, William W., author. | Feldman, Steven R., author. | Ahn, Christine (Christine S.), author. | Lewallen, Robin, author.
Title: Dermatology : illustrated clinical cases / William W. Huang, Steven Feldman, Christine Ahn, Robin S. Lewallen.
Other titles: Illustrated clinical cases.
Description: Boca Raton : CRC Press, [2016] | Series: Illustrated clinical cases
Identifiers: LCCN 2016020962 | ISBN 9781498722889 (pbk. : alk. paper)
Subjects: | MESH: Skin Diseases--diagnosis | Skin Diseases--therapy | Diagnosis, Differential | Case Reports
Classification: LCC RL74 | NLM WR 141 | DDC 616.5--dc23
LC record available at https://lccn.loc.gov/2016020962

Visit the Taylor & Francis Web site at
http://www.taylorandfrancis.com

and the CRC Press Web site at
http://www.crcpress.com

MIX
Paper from responsible sources
FSC
www.fsc.org
FSC® C011748

CONTENTS

Disorders of pigmentation

Neoplasms of the skin

Infections

Drug-related cutaneous disorders

Congenital lesions and lesions of newborns

Genodermatoses

Photodermatologic disorders

Skin findings from external or physical agents

PREFACE

The specialty of dermatology encompasses the medical and surgical treatment of disorders of the hair, skin and nails. Being the largest and most visible organ, physicians of every discipline will encounter patients with dermatologic conditions. In fact, most skin conditions are treated by non-dermatologists. Therefore, it is important for all providers of patient care to have some familiarity with dermatology.

This series of illustrated clinical cases looks to highlight many common and several uncommon dermatologic conditions that one may find in clinical practice. With over 3000 distinct clinical entities, skin conditions can be congenital, inflammatory, autoimmune, autoinflammatory, neoplastic, cosmetic, psychogenic, neuropathic, infectious, paraneoplastic, allergic or idiopathic in nature. Presented in short vignettes with associated images, questions and explanations, the reader will be able to rapidly review the pertinent key facts or 'pearls' from each case. By no means is this book meant to be comprehensive, but rather a companion for ongoing and continuing medical education.

AUTHORS

William W. Huang, MD, MPH, FAAD, is an assistant professor and program director at the Department of Dermatology, School of Medicine, Wake Forest University in Winston-Salem, North Carolina. His clinical and research interests include public health sciences research, complex medical dermatology, dermatologic manifestations of internal disease and autoimmune connective tissue/bullous disorders.

Steven R. Feldman, MD, PhD, is a professor of dermatology, pathology, and public health sciences at Wake Forest Baptist Medical Center in Winston-Salem, North Carolina. He directs the Center for Dermatology Research, a health services research centre whose mission is to improve the care of patients with skin disease. His chief clinical interest is psoriasis and chief research interest is patients' adherence to treatment.

Christine S. Ahn, MD, is a first-year dermatology resident at Wake Forest Baptist Medical Center. Her interests include cost-efficacy in delivering healthcare and inpatient dermatology.

Robin S. Lewallen, MD, is a third-year dermatology resident and co-chief resident at Wake Forest Baptist Medical Center. Her interests include the education of patients and medical professionals as well as implementation of technology to improve patient outcomes.

PAPULOSQUAMOUS AND ECZEMATOUS DISORDERS

CASE 1

Atopic dermatitis

QUESTION 1

An 11-year-old girl presents to the pediatric dermatology clinic as a referral for a persistently itchy rash that involves the face, neck, trunk and extremities. She has been treated by her pediatrician for atopic dermatitis (AD). The pediatrician has been treating the areas with topical hydrocortisone 2.5% cream, which has not helped control the symptoms. Her mother states that despite using generous emollients and hydrocortisone, the girl scratches rigorously at night and is unable to concentrate during school due to pruritus. She has a past medical history of moderate intermittent asthma and allergic rhinitis, and her mother reports a strong history of asthma on her side of the family without any dermatologic issues. On physical examination, there is extensive generalized xerosis of the skin with areas of eczematous lichenified plaques, many with secondary excoriations and hypopigmentation (1).

1

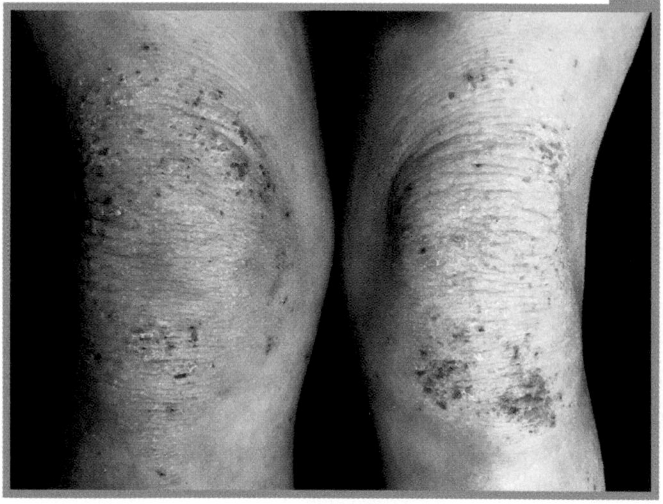

i. What is the pathogenesis of atopic dermatitis?

ii. What are the 'atopic stigmata'?

iii. What treatments are on the therapeutic ladder for atopic dermatitis?

Answer 1

i. Atopic dermatitis also commonly known as eczema, is a common chronic inflammatory disorder of the skin, with a prevalence of up to 30% in children and 10% in adults. Atopic dermatitis is thought to be caused by a combination of genetic and environmental factors. There are two sets of genes that have been implicated: (1) genes encoding epidermal proteins such as filaggrin (*FLG*) and serine protease inhibitor LETKI (*SPINK5*) and (2) genes encoding immunologic proteins such as high-affinity IgE receptors (*FCER1A*), toll-like receptor-2 (*TLR-2*) and different interleukins (*IL4, IL5, IL12B, IL13*), among others. Ichthyosis vulgaris, which is an autosomal semidominant disorder of the skin caused by a mutation in *FLG*, is seen in up to 15% of patients with AD.

Due to genetic factors, patients with atopic dermatitis have an impaired epidermal barrier that is characterized by epidermal barrier dysfunction and increased transepidermal water loss as a result of an altered stratum corneum.

ii. Atopic stigmata are associated features observed in patients with atopic dermatitis. One of the most important cutaneous features observed in patients with atopic dermatitis is xerosis, characterized by dry skin with fine scale, often worse during the winter. Xerosis promotes pruritus, which can lead to inflammation through the release of proinflammatory cytokines by keratinocytes due to scratching.

Additional stigmata include palmar hyperlinearity, white dermatographism, periorbital darkening, pityriasis alba, infraorbital folds (Dennie–Morgan lines), hypodense lateral eyebrows (Hertoghe's sign) and low hairline.

iii. Given the extent and areas of involvement, more potent topical steroids would be appropriate for this patient based on the therapeutic ladder for atopic dermatitis. Triamcinolone 0.1% is appropriate for use on most areas of the skin, excluding the skin folds and face, whereas thicker lichenified plaques can be treated with topical corticosteroids with high or very high potency such as fluocinonide or clobetasol, respectively. In addition to topical steroids, topical calcineurin inhibitors (tacrolimus, pimecrolimus) have demonstrated efficacy in the treatment of AD in prospective controlled trials. Adjunctive therapies include dilute bleach baths, oral antihistamines for antipruritic and sedative effects, cool mist room vaporizers and antibacterial soaps.

Other potential treatments include narrowband UV therapy, cyclosporine, azathioprine, methotrexate and mycophenolate mofetil. The use of systemic corticosteroids should be limited because other agents have a more favourable long-term side-effect profile.

CASE 2

Contact dermatitis

QUESTION 2

A 79-year-old woman presents to a dermatology clinic with a painful, itchy rash on her hand and wrist. The patient is visiting her daughter from South America and reports that while cooking, she sustained burns to the hand and wrist when she came into contact with a hot surface. She attempted to treat the areas with multiple over-the-counter topical medications. She cannot recall what she used but reports using various old antiseptics and ointments she brought from South America. However, her burn wounds have worsened and she has developed increased pain, swelling, erythema and intense pruritus at the sites of the wound. On examination there are well-demarcated scaly orange-red plaques on the medial hand and wrist with superficial fissures (2).

2

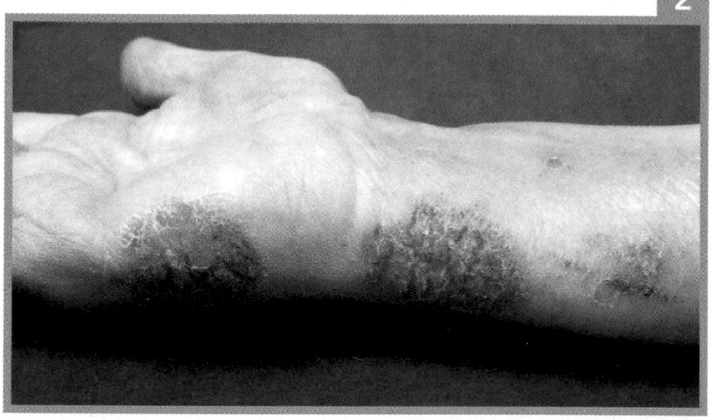

i. What is the diagnosis and the most likely causative material?

ii. What is the name of the syndrome that can result from ingestion of this material?

Answer 2

i. The patient presents with a localized rash around an area of compromised skin barrier, consistent with allergic contact dermatitis. There are various topical agents, such as topical neomycin or fragrance in soaps or moisturizers, that can lead to contact dermatitis. The culprit agent in this patient's rash is merbromin, a topical antiseptic composed of organomercuric disodium salt that is used for minor cuts and burns. Although it is available in many countries, it is no longer available in the United States due to its mercury content. However, patients from other countries may continue to use merbromin. The agent stains the skin red when it is applied, leading to contact dermatitis that has a characteristic orange-red hue.

ii. The systemic ingestion of products containing mercury can lead to baboon syndrome. This occurs after initial sensitization through skin contact, followed by systemic exposure. Classic baboon syndrome was originally seen with mercury, nickel and ampicillin. The rash often involves skin flexures, but characteristically involves a well-defined erythematous area of the buttocks and upper inner thighs. Patch testing can be useful to identify the causative agent and withdrawal of the agent will lead to spontaneous resolution. Topical steroids can be used to reduce erythema and discomfort associated with pruritus.

CASE 3

Psoriasis

QUESTION 3

A 47-year-old man presents to the dermatology clinic with a pruritic scaly eruption on his body. He states that he began developing similar lesions in his 30s, but over the last several years developed more widespread disease. He notes that his disease is quiescent over the summer months and tends to flare during the winter. He has tried over-the-counter anti-itch creams and other moisturizers without success. His father had a similar skin disease. On examination, there are well-demarcated erythematous plaques with overlying thick adherent scale distributed over the extensor arms and legs, lower back, buttocks and periumbilical region, with a total body surface area (BSA) of involvement around 10% (3). Review of systems is positive for stiffness in the hands, more noticeable in the morning for at least 1–2 hours and improving throughout the day.

3

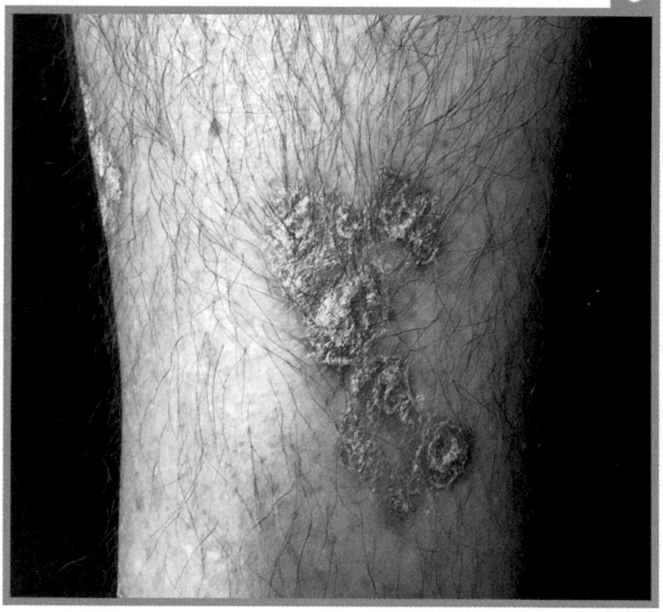

i. What is the most likely diagnosis?

ii. What are key pathogenic factors and triggering factors in this disease?

iii. What is the next best step in the management of this patient?

Answer 3

i. Based on the patient's history and clinical presentation, the most likely diagnosis is the chronic plaque psoriasis variant of psoriasis vulgaris, a chronic immune-mediated inflammatory skin disorder. Psoriasis is a relatively common disease, estimated in up to 2% of the world's population. Although it can present at nearly any age, the most common ages of onset are bimodal, with peaks observed in the third and sixth decades of life. A positive family history of psoriasis can be seen in 30%–90% of patients. Specific human leukocyte antigens (HLA) such as HLA-Cw6 have also been strongly linked to psoriasis, particularly early onset disease.

Chronic plaque psoriasis is characterized classically by the presence of well-demarcated erythematous plaques with a thick 'micaceous' overlying scale. Common sites affected are the scalp, elbows, knees and presacrum.

ii. Although the pathogenesis has not been completely elucidated, a combination of abnormal T-cell activation and abnormal keratinocytes are known to play important roles. Potential triggering factors in psoriasis include physical trauma (also known as the Köebner phenomenon), infections such as streptococcal pharyngitis, stress and medications such as lithium, beta-blockers and nonsteroidal anti-inflammatory drugs, among others.

iii. Although the patient's cutaneous manifestations alone could be managed with topical medications, the presence of symptoms such as joint symptoms should raise concern for psoriatic arthritis, which is a seronegative, HLAB27-associated arthritis seen in up to 30% of patients with psoriasis. In patients with psoriatic arthritis, there is an increased level of tumor necrosis factor-alpha (TNF-α) within the synovium and serum and even with mild or absent skin findings, treatment with systemic agents is indicated. Treatment options for psoriatic arthritis include methotrexate, apremilast, TNF-α antagonists such as adalimumab, infliximab and etanercept and other biologics such as certolizumab pegol, golimumab and ustekinumab. If joint disease is suspected, a referral to a rheumatologist for evaluation is indicated.

CASE 4

Lichen planus

QUESTION 4

A 64-year-old woman presents to the dermatology clinic for evaluation of itchy bumps on the hands and wrists. The symptoms have been present for several months and seem to be spreading. On examination, there are multiple violaceous, polygonal flat-topped papules, some with overlying lacy white reticulations (4). There are no intraoral or genital lesions. Her past medical history is notable for hepatitis C infection.

4

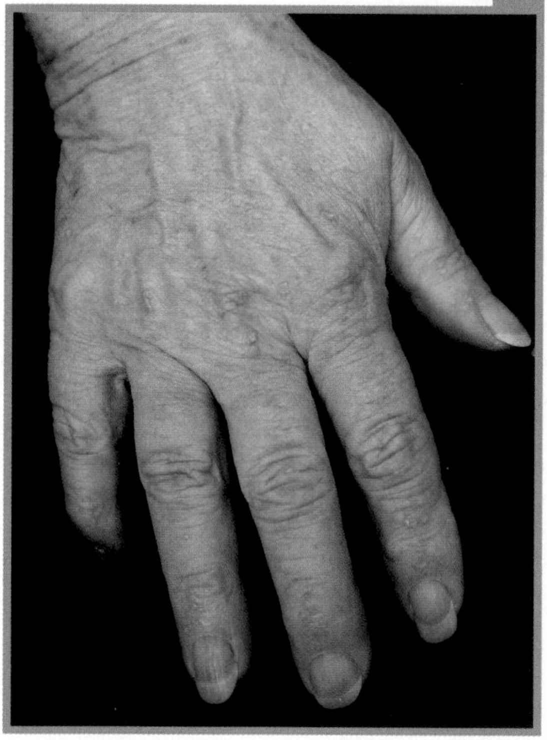

i. What is the diagnosis?

ii. What are the major clinical variants and their characteristic features?

iii. If this condition were due to a drug, what are the most common culprit medications?

Answer 4

i. The patient presents with classic features of lichen planus (LP), an idiopathic inflammatory disease that affects the skin and mucous membranes. It is most often seen in adults but can be seen in infants and children. Although the pathogenesis has not been completely elucidated, it is thought to be a T-cell-mediated autoimmune process that leads to damage of basal keratinocytes. There are some theories that exogenous antigens may play a role in LP. In Japanese and Mediterranean populations, an association has been observed between hepatitis C virus infections and LP.

ii. The characteristic lesion of lichen planus is a flat-topped, polygonal, violaceous papule. Overlying the papule, a network of lacy white reticulations can often be observed and is referred to as 'Wickham's striae'. Lichen planopilaris is a clinical variant of LP, which involves the hair follicle and can lead to a scarring alopecia of the scalp. Lichen planus of the nails can be seen alone or with other clinical variants. The classic nail findings of LP are lateral thinning, longitudinal ridging, fissuring, scarring and formation of dorsal pterygium. Oral LP can be seen in various forms but the most common form is the reticular pattern, which is characterized by white lacy lines on bilateral buccal mucosa and is occasionally associated with desquamative gingivitis. Vulvovaginal LP is most commonly erosive and can lead to scarring.

iii. Drugs can be responsible for cutaneous eruptions that appear similar or identical to LP. These drug reactions are described as 'lichen planus–like' or 'lichenoid'. Drugs that are commonly implicated in producing lichenoid drug eruptions include antihypertensives such as enalapril, captopril, labetalol, propranolol, diuretics such as hydrochlorothiazide, antimalarials such as hydroxychloroquine and chloroquine and biologic drugs including etanercept and infliximab.

CASE 5

Pityriasis rubra pilaris

QUESTION 5

A 54-year-old male presents to the dermatology office as a referral for the rapid onset of erythroderma. The changes initially presented on his head and neck. He was treated for seborrheic dermatitis with ketoconazole 2% shampoo. Despite treatment, the rash spread caudally over the next few weeks, with 90% BSA involvement. He feels that he is worse with exposure to UV light. On physical examination, there are confluent salmon-coloured thin plaques with islands of sparing. There is also follicular hyperkeratosis giving the skin a nutmeg grater appearance (5a). The palms and soles have an orange-red waxy keratoderma (5b); however, the nails appear normal without pits, onycholysis or oil drops.

5a

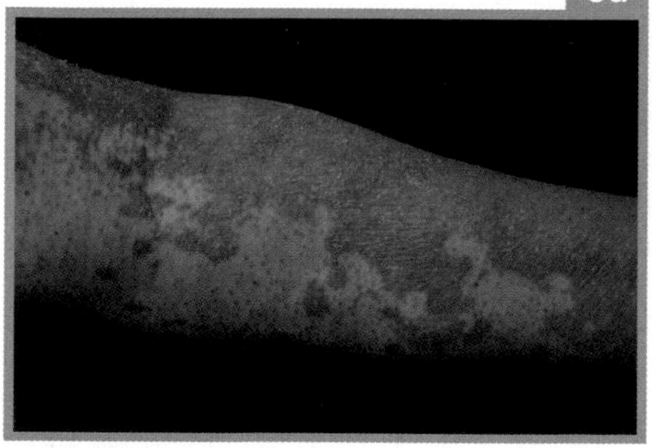

5b

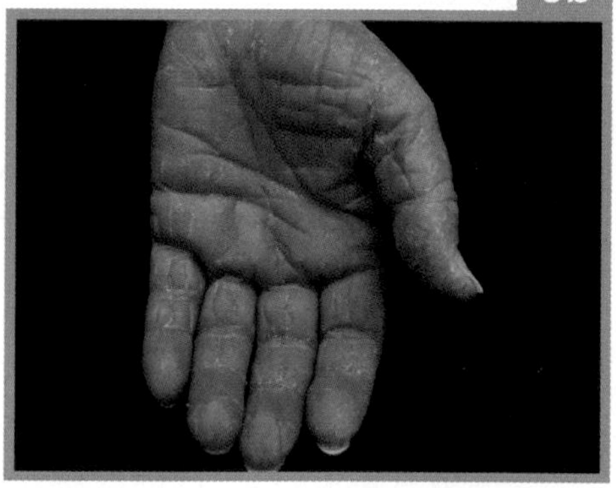

i. There are five types of this condition; which is the most common in adults? In children?

ii. How long does this presentation typically last?

Answer 5

i. Pityriasis rubra pilaris (PRP) is a papulosquamous disorder seen in all ages and genders. There is a bimodal age distribution with the first peak seen during the first and second decades and the second peak during the sixth decade. There are five subtypes, with the classic adult form, type I, being the most common comprising 55% of cases. The classic adult form presents with a cephalocaudal spread of red-orange plaques with islands of sparing, perifollicular keratotic papules and a waxy palmoplantar keratoderma. The most common subtype in children (type IV), comprising 25% of all cases of PRP, is the circumscribed juvenile form, which presents with disease limited to the elbows and knees most often with a prepubertal onset. There is a classic juvenile variant, type III, which presents with the same clinical findings as type I, but this presentation is only seen in 10% of cases.

ii. This case presents a patient with classic adult type I disease. The majority of cases clear within 3 years even without treatment. There are treatments available that can provide temporizing relief while awaiting spontaneous resolution. Classic treatments include oral retinoids, such as acitretin or immunosuppressants, such as methotrexate, corticosteroids, cyclosporine and azathioprine. Less toxic regimens are recommended for the classic juvenile form given the high rates of spontaneous resolution within 3 years without treatment. The circumscribed juvenile variant, type IV, has a variable course and the atypical adult, type II and atypical juvenile, type V, tend to have a chronic course.

CASE 6

Pityriasis lichenoides et varioliformis acuta

QUESTION 6

A 12-year-old boy presents to the pediatric dermatology office as a referral for the abrupt onset of widespread erythematous crusted papules. His mother states that he has had vesicles off and on since 7 years old without a definitive diagnosis being given. The skin changes come up in April and usually resolves by September. The lesions are intensely pruritic. He has been seen by his pediatrician and treated with desoximetasone 0.05% cream without resolution of his symptoms. On physical examination, there are widespread erythematous and heme-crusted papules some with superficial ulceration. Some of these are varioliform and in various stages of healing (6a, b).

6a

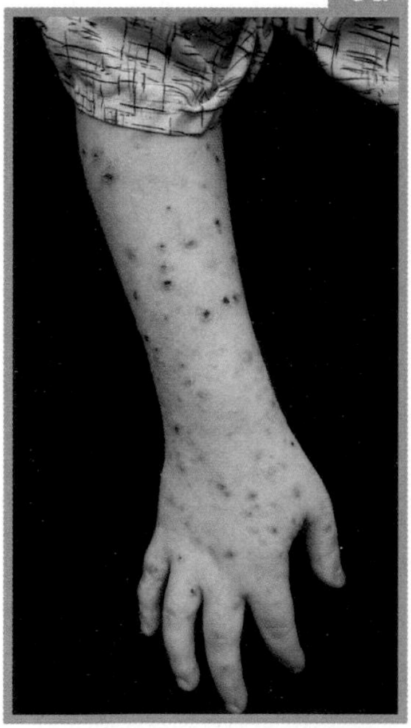

6b

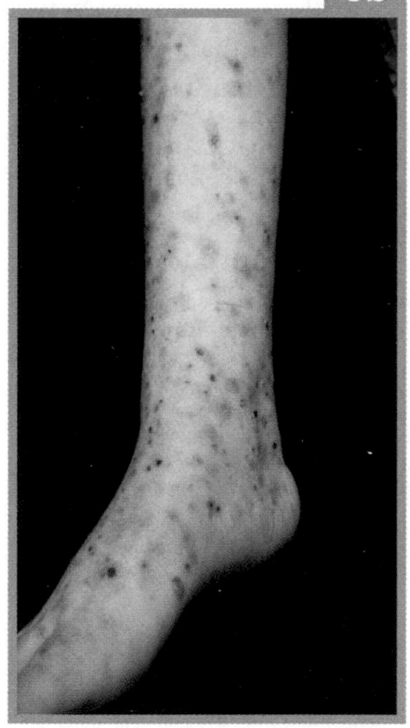

i. What is the diagnosis?

ii. Are recurrences common or rare in this condition?

iii. If a patient with these skin changes also developed systemic manifestations (malaise, fever, lymphadenopathy, arthritis, bacteremia and/or mucosal involvement) what rare disorder should be considered in the differential?

Answer 6

i. Pityriasis lichenoides et varioliformis acuta (PLEVA) formerly known as Mucha–Habermann disease is a papulosquamous disorder that primarily affects the pediatric population with a male predominance. A skin biopsy is confirmatory and often shows parakeratosis, interface dermatitis, necrosis and extravasation of red blood cells. The main differential includes varicella, viral exanthem, drug eruption, lymphomatoid papulosis, vasculitis, secondary syphilis, guttate psoriasis, pityriasis rosea, lichen planus and pityriasis lichenoides chronica.

ii. Recurrent episodes of PLEVA are common and should be discussed with patients and their parents. Recurrent episodes can occur for months to years. First line treatments for this condition include topical corticosteroids, topical coal tar preparations, oral antibiotics and phototherapy. Antibiotics, such as erythromycin, are selected for their anti-inflammatory properties and antibiotic course duration is usually for several months.

iii. Rarely, PLEVA can be associated with systemic manifestations. This presentation is known as febrile ulceronecrotic Mucha–Habermann disease (FUMHD). This febrile variant is associated with increased levels of TNF-α. Once the diagnosis of FUMHD is established and infection has been excluded, treatment options include systemic corticosteroids, intravenous immunoglobulin (IVIg) or cyclosporine.

URTICARIAS AND ERYTHEMAS

CASE 7

Urticaria

QUESTION 7

A 32-year-old woman presented to the emergency department (ED) with acute onset hives. While in the ED she was treated with intramuscular methylprednisolone and intravenous diphenhydramine with complete resolution of her symptoms. Eight weeks after her ED visit, she continued to have intermittent hives more than 5 days a week. The hives were unresponsive to loratadine 10 mg daily so she decided to visit a dermatologist. On examination, there are numerous annular and geographic edematous plaques on the inner thighs and upper back (7). Upon further questioning, she denies worsening with pressure, cold, heat, water or exercise.

7

i. What is the most accurate diagnosis?

ii. What is the most likely cause?

iii. What type of exogenous physical stimuli can cause this condition?

iv. What are the potential pharmacologic treatments available and what medications should be avoided in these patients?

Answer 7

i. Based on the patient's clinical presentation and course, the most accurate diagnosis is chronic urticaria, which is defined as continuous urticaria occurring for over 6 weeks, at least twice weekly while off treatment.

Urticaria is a term used to describe recurrent wheals that are pruritic, pink swellings of the superficial dermis lasting less than 24 hours. In contrast, angioedema is a swelling that occurs deeper in the dermis and subcutaneous tissue and may affect the mouth and bowel. Cutaneous findings can be minimal or absent and can last up to several days.

ii. The patient most likely has an 'ordinary' or spontaneous chronic urticaria, which makes up about 60% of all cases of chronic urticaria. Among the causes, the most likely is idiopathic, followed by autoimmune, infection-related or pseudoallergic causes. Among the remaining 40% of chronic urticarias, approximately 35% are physical or inducible urticaria, which are induced by exogenous physical stimuli and 5% are due to a vasculitis process, characterized by leukocytoclastic vasculitis.

iii. Physical or inducible urticarias can be divided into broad categories based on the type of stimulus, including mechanical stimulus, temperature changes and sweating or stress. Examples of urticaria due to mechanical stimuli include dermatographism, which manifests as linear wheals occurring at sites of friction or shearing force, and delayed pressure urticaria, which presents as wheals at sites of sustained pressure to the skin. Urticaria due to temperature changes can be seen with heat or cold exposure. Urticaria due to sweating or stress includes cholinergic urticaria, which occurs within 15 minutes of sweat-inducing stimuli, and exercise-induced anaphylaxis, which can occur within minutes of exercise.

iv. Antihistamines are the first-line medication for most patients with urticaria and should be taken on a daily basis rather than when symptomatic. Second-line medications for chronic or physical urticaria can be considered when antihistamines alone do not control symptoms. Some second-line targeted therapies include prednisone, epinephrine, montelukast, colchicine and sulfasalazine, particularly for delayed pressure urticaria. Non-steroidal anti-inflammatory drugs (NSAIDs) should be avoided in patients with urticaria.

CASE 8

Dermatographism

QUESTION 8

A 36-year-old woman was recently evaluated by her dermatologist for a scabies infestation. She and her family were successfully treated with permethrin cream 5%. After initial resolution of symptoms, she presents with ongoing pruritus, particularly around her bra straps, that is worse in the evenings. On examination, gentle scraping on the back with a tongue depressor in a linear fashion results in erythema with raised wheals in the distribution of the scraping (8).

8

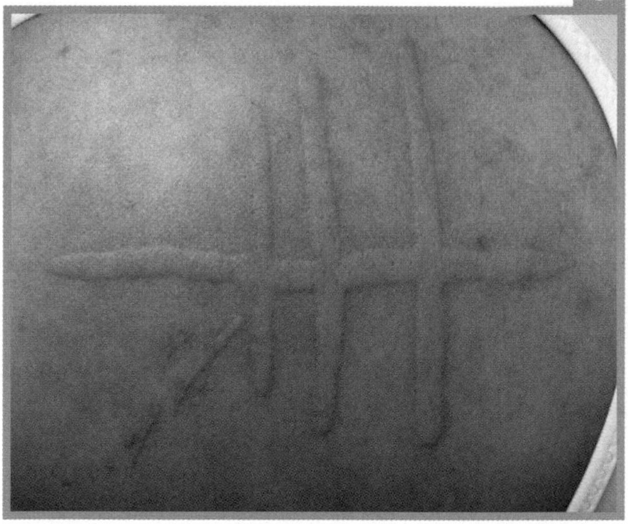

i. What is the diagnosis?

ii. What are some of the first- and second-line therapeutic options for this condition?

Answer 8

i. The patient presents with symptomatic dermatographism, which is the most common type of physical urticaria. It is not associated with systemic disease, atopy, food allergy or autoimmunity and can be seen in patients after scabies infestation or with a penicillin allergy. Symptomatic dermatographism is most commonly see in young adults and is characterized by the appearance of wheals at sites of minor scratches, trauma or friction on the skin. Patients often complain of worsening of symptoms at night-time, but lesions typically resolve over the course of hours.

ii. The first-line treatment for symptomatic dermatographism is antihistamine therapy. Daily therapy with second-generation H_1 antihistamines is recommended. The addition of H_2 antagonists may have benefit in patients with chronic urticaria, although there is limited evidence to support combining H_1 and H_2 antihistamines. H_2 histamines should not be used as monotherapy, as they have no effect on histamine-induced pruritus.

Second-line therapies can be used in patients who do not respond well to antihistamines. Some second-line medications that have been studied in retrospective studies or large case studies include oral prednisone as a burst therapy for severe exacerbations and intramuscular or subcutaneous epinephrine for cases with angioedema or anaphylactic symptoms. Doxepin is a tricyclic antidepressant with additional H_1 and H_2 antihistamine properties that produces sedative and anticholinergic effects, which may be used in patients with chronic urticaria. Additional agents that have been reported in small case series or case reports include montelukast, colchicine and sulfasalazine.

CASE 9

Erythema multiforme

QUESTION 9

A 29-year-old man presents to the ED with a generalized rash that began on the arms and chest and spread to involve the palms, face and back. He was seen by his primary care physician 5 days ago for the development of cold sores and was prescribed oral acyclovir. He denies treatment with any other new medications and has no other medical problems. On examination, there are erythematous, raised papules on the face, back and extremities with a violaceous hue, some with a targetoid appearance (9a, b). Other than a resolving herpetic blister on the vermillion border of the lower lip, there are no signs of mucosal or intraoral involvement.

9a

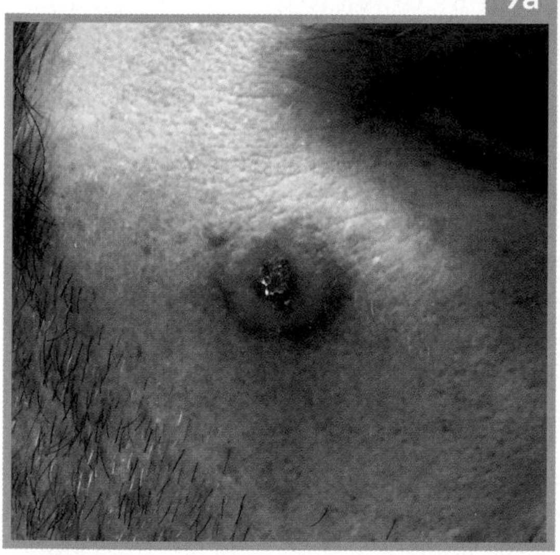

9b

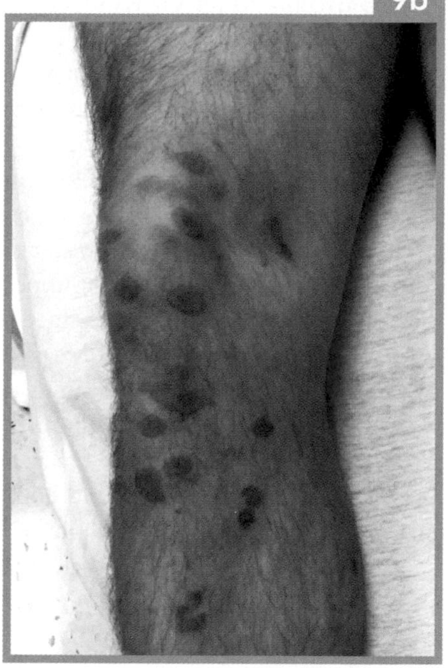

i. What is the most likely diagnosis? What is the most likely causative agent?

ii. What are other less common causative agents?

iii. What are classic histologic features of this rash?

iv. What are the associated human leukocyte antigens (HLAs) (if any)?

Answer 9

i. Based on the lack of systemic symptoms or mucosal involvement, this patient's presentation is most consistent with erythema multiforme (EM) minor. EM is an acute, self-limited condition characterized by the abrupt onset of fixed red papules that may evolve into targetoid lesions. It can be classified as EM minor or EM major; the two forms are distinguished by the presence of severe mucosal involvement and systemic symptoms in EM major. Although historically considered to be within a spectrum with Stevens–Johnson syndrome (SJS) based on presentation and mucosal involvement, the two are distinct entities.

The most common precipitating factor in EM is infection, accounting for approximately 90% of cases. Among viral infections, the most common is herpes simplex virus (HSV)-1 or -2, as was the case in this vignette. Other viral infections include parapoxvirus (orf disease), vaccinia (smallpox vaccine), varicella-zoster virus, adenovirus and Epstein–Barr virus. Common bacterial infections that precipitate EM are *Mycoplasma pneumonia, Chlamydophila psittaci, Salmonella* and *Mycobacterium tuberculosis.* Occasionally, fungal infections such as *Histoplasma capsulatum* can be the causative agent.

The characteristic skin lesion of EM is a well-demarcated, round, target-shaped papule. Atypical papular target lesions in EM are round, edematous and often have a poorly defined border or lack distinctly demarcated rings of clearing. EM typically favours the upper extremities in a symmetric distribution and often involves the palms, face and trunk. Mucosal lesions are vesiculobullous and develop into painful erosions, usually on the buccal mucosa and lips. Uncommonly, they can involve the ocular and genital mucosae. The presence of systemic symptoms supports the diagnosis of EM major. The most common symptoms reported are fever, arthralgia and occasionally pulmonary symptoms. Rarely, renal, hepatic and hematologic abnormalities occur. The skin lesions of EM appear suddenly and evolve over 72 hours. For most individuals, EM is self-limited and resolves over 2 weeks without sequelae. However, patients with HSV-associated EM can have recurrent disease.

ii. Drugs are a less common precipitating factor in EM. The primary culprit medications that have been identified in the setting of EM are NSAIDs, sulfonamides, anticonvulsants, aminopenicillins and allopurinol. Certain exposures, such as to poison ivy, can uncommonly trigger the development of EM. In rare cases, EM can occur in the setting of systemic diseases such as inflammatory bowel disease, lupus erythematosus and Behçet's disease.

iii. The classic histologic findings of EM are the presence of spongiosis and focal vacuolar degeneration of basal keratinocytes with dermal edema and perivascular lymphocytic infiltrates.

iv. There is no clearly defined genetic predisposition for the development of EM, though small studies have shown association with HLA-DQw3 (especially for HSV-associated EM), HLA-DRw53 and HLA-Aw33.

VESICULOBULLOUS DISORDER

CASE 10

Bullous pemphigoid

QUESTION 10

A 74-year-old man with a history of congestive heart failure presents to the emergency department with an itchy rash with blisters on his trunk and arms. He reports that he has had a 2-month history of intractable pruritus prior to the formation of blisters. He had been evaluated initially by his family practitioner with non-specific skin findings including scattered urticarial papules, eczema and associated excoriations. He had been treated empirically for scabies with permethrin 5% cream without improvement. On examination, there are multiple excoriated scaly papules and plaques, and several tense bullae on the trunk and arms (10a, b). A complete blood count (CBC) reveals peripheral eosinophilia.

10a

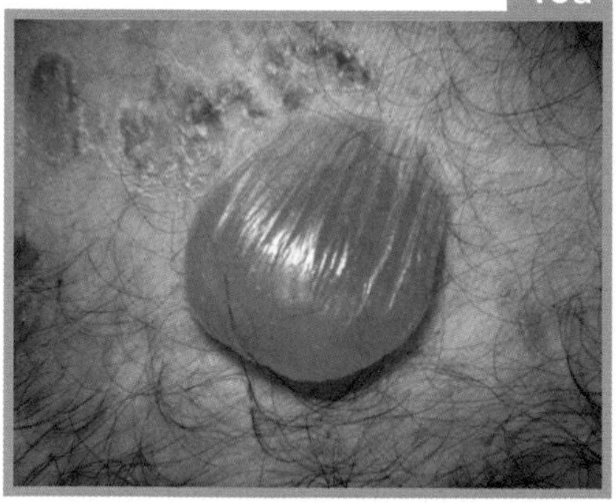

10b

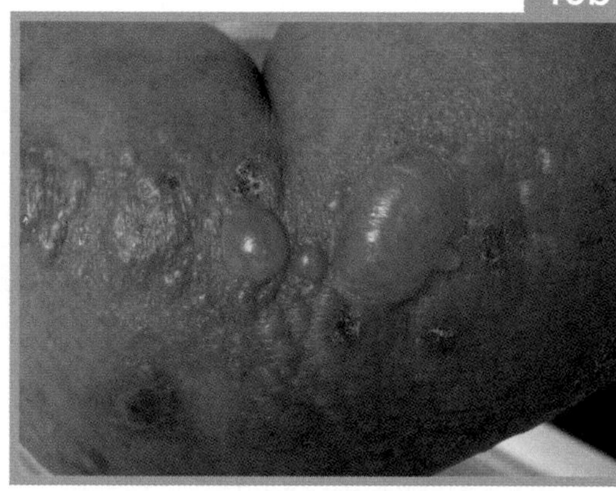

i. What is the diagnosis and on what site(s) should a biopsy be performed?

ii. What treatments are available for this condition?

iii. What other tests are indicated in the work-up of this condition?

Answer 10

i. This patient presents with bullous pemphigoid (BP), an autoimmune subepidermal bullous disease that is usually seen in patients older than 60 years of age. BP can present with a non-specific, non-bullous prodromal phase with a wide range of symptoms including pruritus, eczematous papules and/or urticarial lesions that may persist for weeks or months. Particularly in elderly patients, pruritus is common. The non-bullous phase often goes undiagnosed and patients may be empirically treated for other conditions that can cause intense pruritus such as scabies or eczema. In the bullous phase, vesicles and bullae form on normal and erythematous skin and favour flexural areas and the lower trunk in a symmetrical distribution. Although mucosal involvement is rare, oral cavity involvement is seen in 10%–30% of patients and peripheral eosinophilia is seen in up to 50% of patients. In the elderly, BP can be associated with significant morbidity and mortality, with an estimated mortality rate between 10% and 40% within the first year.

Skin biopsies with hematoxylin and eosin (H&E) staining and direct immunofluorescence (DIF) will confirm the diagnosis of BP. On H&E staining, BP classically shows a subepidermal blister containing fibrin, eosinophils and mononuclear cells, and an upper dermal inflammatory infiltrate composed of eosinophils and mononuclear cells. For DIF, biopsies should be taken from perilesional, uninvolved skin. A positive DIF will demonstrate fine, linear, continuous deposits of IgG and/or complement 3 (C3) along the basement membrane.

ii. The treatment with systemic steroids is indicated for patients with generalized disease. The recommended daily dose of prednisone ranges from 0.5 to 1 mg/kg/day. Steroids should be tapered slowly over 6–9 months or longer to minimize the risk of disease rebound. Recent studies have emphasized the role of potent topical corticosteroids such as clobetasol propionate even in generalized disease, due to similar efficacy and fewer systemic adverse effects with long-term use. This option should be considered in patients with multiple co-morbidities in which the risk of systemic corticosteroids outweighs the benefits.

There is limited evidence supporting the use of other immunosuppressive drugs. Agents such as azathioprine, mycophenolate mofetil, methotrexate, chlorambucil and cyclophosphamide are considered second-line.

iii. BP can be associated with malignancies including lymphoproliferative disorders and cancer of the digestive tract, urinary bladder and lung. Although the older age of patients with BP likely contributes to this association, patients should undergo appropriate age-related screening tests during the work-up of new onset BP.

Other significant associations include trauma, Parkinson's disease, inflammatory bowel disease and rheumatoid arthritis. Drug-induced BP has been linked to diuretics, neuroleptics, antibiotics, potassium iodide, gold, analgesics and captopril. Careful drug history and discontinuation of any potential culprit medications is essential.

CASE 11

Pemphigus vegetans

QUESTION 11

A previously healthy 56-year-old woman presents to a clinic with a 4-month history of odynophagia and hemoptysis. She first noticed ulcerations of her oral cavity and lips but within weeks developed similar ulcerations of her external genitalia and inguinal folds. She can now only tolerate liquids secondary to severe pain with swallowing. Over the past 3 weeks, her symptoms have worsened and the ulcerations have spread. On examination, she has involvement of 10% of her body surface area including lips, oral mucosa, internal nares, scalp, face, neck, trunk, proximal extremities and external genitalia with shallow ulcerations that are Nikolsky's sign positive (11a, b).

11a

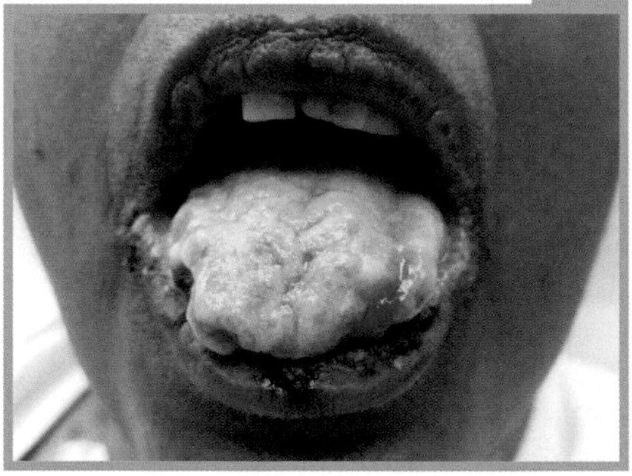

11b

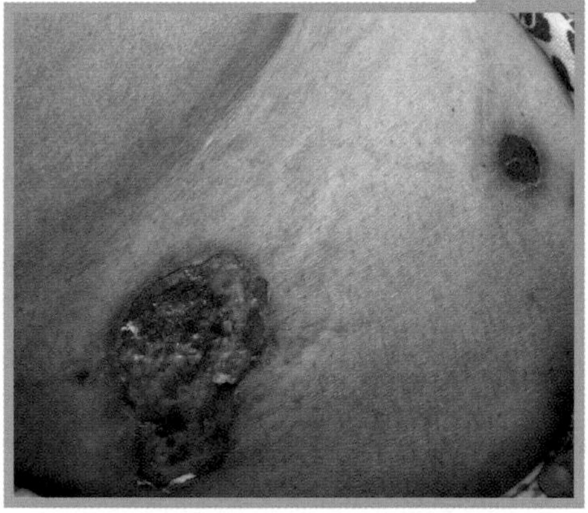

i. What is the most likely diagnosis?

ii. What is an important differential diagnosis for this condition and how can the two entities be distinguished?

iii. What is the best treatment modality?

Answer 11

i. This patient presents with pemphigus vegetans, a rare variant of pemphigus vulgaris (PV), comprising, 2%–7% of cases of PV. It occurs predominantly in middle-aged women, but can be seen in all ages, including children. There are two clinical subtypes of pemphigus vegetans: (1) Neumann and (2) Hallopeau. This patient's clinical presentation and appearance of lesions are consistent with the Neumann subtype of pemphigus vegetans, which is more common than the Hallopeau subtype. It is characterized by an eruption of flaccid bullae that erode and form secondary hypertrophic papillated plaques. In the Hallopeau subtype, patients present with polycyclic pustules that erode and evolve into verrucous and papillomatous vegetations. Lesions of both subtypes have a predilection for intertriginous regions, and oral mucosa involvement is present in almost all reported cases of pemphigus vegetans. The patient in this case demonstrates a cerebriform tongue, characterized by sulci and gyri on the dorsum of the tongue. Other special sites for pemphigus vegetans include the vermillion border of the lips, the angle of the mouth and around the nares. Patients rarely may present with features of both clinical subtypes, either occurring simultaneously or throughout the course of the disease.

Histopathologically, pemphigus vegetans demonstrates epidermal hyperplasia, papillomatosis, acanthosis, and intraepidermal abscesses. Compared with PV, pemphigus vegetans has a more prominent eosinophilic response, microabscess formation, and vesiculation. On DIF, pemphigus vegetans and PV both demonstrate intraepidermal intercellular IgG and/or C3 staining.

ii. An important entity in the differential diagnosis of pemphigus vegetans is pyodermatitis–pyostomatitis vegetans, which shares similar clinical and histological features but is characteristically negative on immunofluorescence testing. In contrast to pemphigus vegetans, pyodermatitis–pyostomatitis vegetans is associated with inflammatory bowel disease, and further laboratory screening is often indicated in patients with this disease.

iii. Similar to PV, first-line treatment for pemphigus vegetans is systemic corticosteroids. In cases where steroids alone do not induce disease remission, adjunctive immunosuppressive agents such as methotrexate, mycophenolate mofetil, azathioprine, cyclosporine and cyclophosphamide are indicated.

CASE 12

Pemphigus foliaceus

QUESTION 12

A 71-year-old woman presents to a dermatology clinic with a scaly, crusted rash on the chest and back. She states that they began to develop as blisters initially, but would burst within a day and leave behind a scaly rash that is mildly painful and pruritic. She denies any recent illness or changes to her personal care products. On examination, there are scattered erythematous and hyperpigmented macules and papules with overlying scale and secondary excoriations on the upper chest and back (12). There is no involvement of the oral or genital mucosa.

12

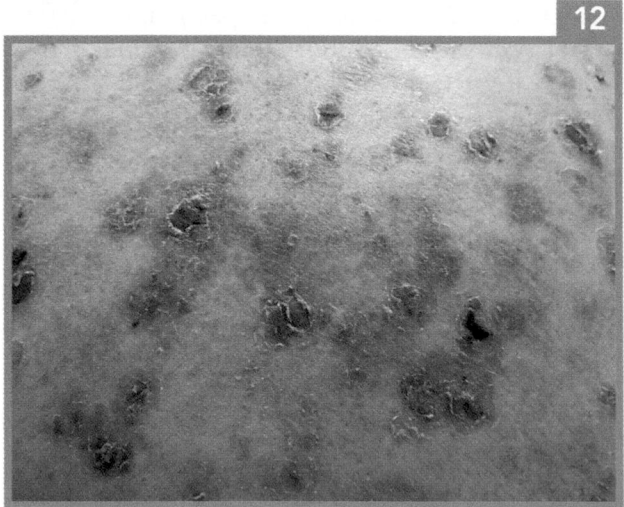

i. What is the most likely diagnosis? What molecule is most likely to be targeted in the pathology of this disease?

ii. What are the characteristic features on histology and immunofluorescence studies? What substrate should be used for indirect immunofluorescence studies?

iii. What is the first-line treatment of choice?

Answer 12

i. The patient's history and the clinical presentation are most consistent with pemphigus foliaceus, a form of pemphigus. In most populations, pemphigus vulgaris is more common than pemphigus foliaceus, except among the populations of Finland, Tunisia and Brazil. Unlike pemphigus vulgaris, pemphigus foliaceus rarely involves the oral mucosa. It is caused by the development of IgG autoantibodies against desmoglein-1 (DSG1), a protein found in desmosomes in the keratinocytes of the skin.

Clinically, patients develop scattered scaly, crusted erosions often distributed on the scalp, face and upper trunk. The primary lesions are vesicles and bullae but are typically so superficial and fragile that the resultant crust and scale are the main findings on examination.

ii. On histopathologic examination, blisters in pemphigus foliaceus demonstrate acantholysis in the upper epidermis, often similar in appearance to that seen in staphylococcal scalded skin syndrome or bullous impetigo. On direct immunofluorescence studies, IgG deposition can be seen on the keratinocyte cell surfaces. Indirect immunofluorescence performed on a guinea pig esophagus can be used to detect anti-DSG1 autoantibodies.

iii. In localized disease, pemphigus foliaceus can be managed with potent topical corticosteroids. For more widespread and active disease, systemic medications such as those used for pemphigus vulgaris are used, including prednisone, mycophenolate mofetil and other immunosuppressants.

CASE 13

Ocular cicatricial pemphigoid

QUESTION 13

A 70-year-old man presents to an ophthalmology clinic with soreness and bilateral eye burning. He has noticed a foreign body sensation and increased crusting around the eyes in the morning. His past medical history is notable only for hypertension. He states that his symptoms began approximately 4 months ago and have worsened over time. On examination, he has an adhesion between the bulbar and palpebral conjunctival surfaces in both lower eyelids (13a, b). He does not have any other skin lesions.

13a

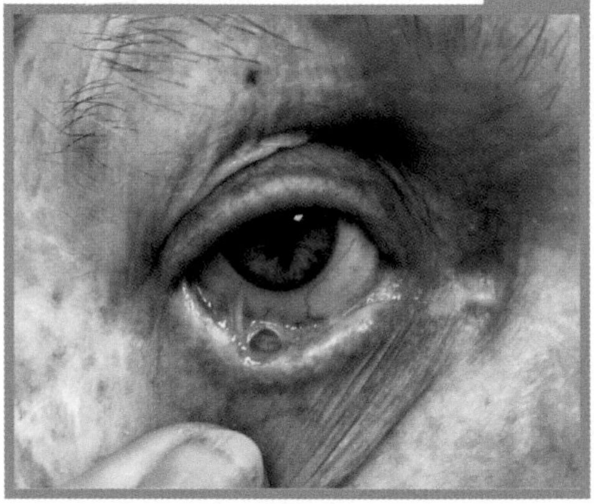

13b

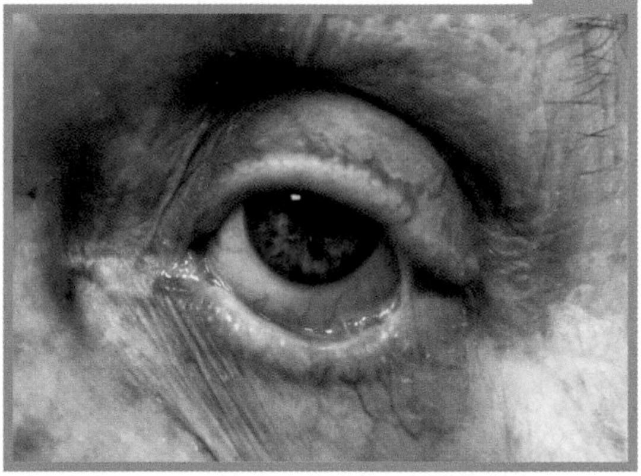

i. What is the diagnosis and what are other clinical features of this disease?

ii. What is the immunogenic haplotype that is associated with this specific disease?

iii. What are the complications of this disease if uncontrolled?

iv. What is the treatment of choice?

Answer 13

i. The presence of symblepharon, or adhesions between the bulbar and palpebral conjunctival surfaces, is suggestive of cicatricial or mucous membrane pemphigoid. Like other forms of pemphigoid, cicatricial pemphigoid is a subepithelial blistering disorder that affects the external mucosal surfaces. The two most common sites of involvement in the cicatricial pemphigoid are the conjunctival and oral mucosae. Conjunctival surfaces are often the only site affected and often start unilaterally and progress to involve both the eyes. Clinically, patients present with non-specific ocular symptoms such as itching, burning, soreness and foreign body sensation associated with inflammation. In cases with oral involvement, a common presentation is a desquamative gingivitis, along with erosions and pain. Other mucosal involvement such as nasopharyngeal, laryngeal, esophageal or anogenital mucosae is relatively rare.

Cutaneous involvement is seen in 25%–30% of patients, most often involving the scalp, face, neck and upper trunk. It is characterized by erythematous plaques within which blisters and erosions occur and recur, leading to scarring and atrophy. The Brunsting-Perry variant is one in which skin lesions are limited to the head and neck region without mucosal involvement. Lesions of the scalp lead to scarring alopecia.

ii. Several studies have shown an association with the specific immunogenic haplotype human leukocyte antigen (HLA-DQw7).

iii. Chronic inflammation on the conjunctiva can lead to scar and symblepharon formation. Fibrosis of the conjunctiva can lead to inwardly angled eyelashes and entropion that can lead to superficial corneal trauma, corneal neovascularization, corneal ulceration and blindness. Complications of nasopharyngeal involvement include adhesions and airway involvement. Laryngeal involvement can be life-threatening, with potential for stenosis-associated dysphagia.

iv. Dapsone is the first-line therapy for oral and cutaneous lesions and is also used for mild ocular disease. For rapidly progressive or severe ocular disease, cyclophosphamide is used, occasionally in combination with oral corticosteroids depending on response to the therapy. Topical treatment can be used for mild to moderate disease.

CASE 14

Friction blister

QUESTION 14

A 56-year-old man presents to the clinic with a painful blister on the great toe. The area was initially erythematous and mildly tender but rapidly developed into a painful, tense blister. He does not have any other blisters on his body but has an erythematous area in a similar distribution on the opposite foot. He reports a lifelong history of frequently developing blisters on his feet and heels. On examination, there is a large tense bulla filled with yellow-red fluid and with minimal erythema, induration or fluctuation (14).

14

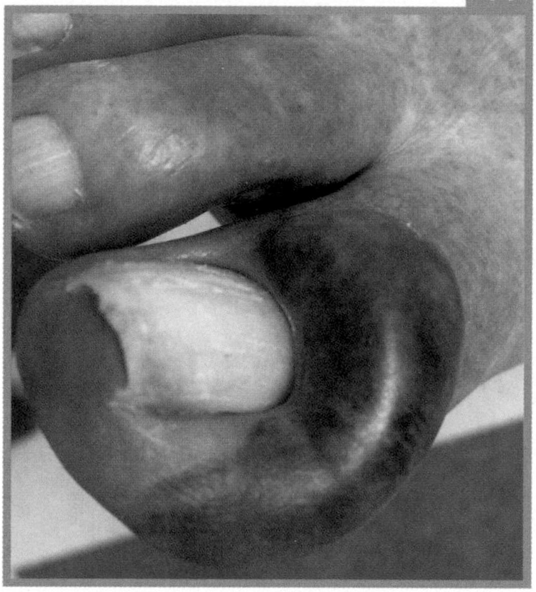

i. What is the most likely diagnosis? What is the most likely cause of this condition?

ii. What underlying systemic diseases may be considered in the context of this condition?

Answer 14

i. This patient has developed a friction blister, which occurs most commonly on the soles and heels. They are the result of repeated frictional shearing force, often due to poor fitting shoes, heat and sweating. The lesions are initially erythematous macules at the sites of contact and develop into bullae with clear or blood-tinged fluid. The blisters are intraepidermal, typically occurring at the level of the stratum spinosum.

ii. Although friction blisters are common in the general population, patients who demonstrate frequent and exaggerated responses to friction should raise the suspicion of a localized variant of epidermolysis bullosa simplex, also known as Weber–Cockayne syndrome. Localized epidermolysis bullosa simplex is inherited in an autosomal dominant manner and is caused by defective keratin 5 or keratin 14 proteins. These diagnoses can be distinguished by histological examination; in contrast to the intraepidermal split featured in friction blisters, epidermolysis bullosa simplex will demonstrate subepidermal separation.

ADNEXAL DISORDERS

CASE 15

Acne vulgaris

QUESTION 15

A 20-year-old man presents to the dermatology office for evaluation of worsening acne. He has struggled with acne since adolescence and has tried numerous topical over-the-counter products containing salicylic acid and benzoyl peroxide and prescription medications including topical clindamycin 1% gel, dapsone gel, topical azelaic acid and a topical retinoid, with only moderate improvement of his acne. He is concerned about the worsening of acne on other parts of his body, including the chest and the back. On examination, there are a few scattered erythematous papules and pustules on the forehead, cheeks and the chin (15a). On the back, there are erythematous papules, pustules, and hyperpigmented papules and scars from prior acne lesions (15b).

15a

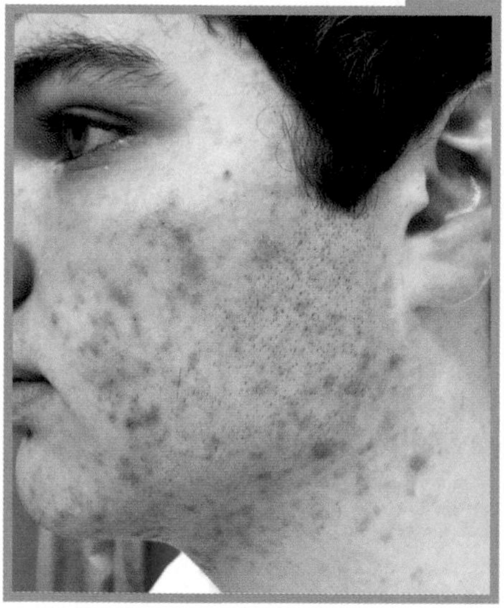

15b

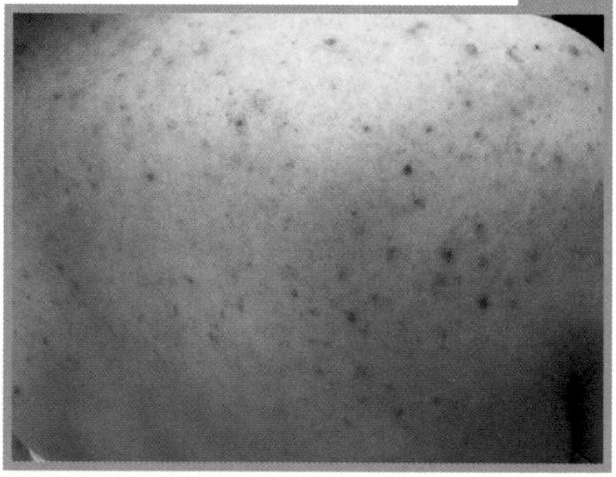

i. What is the pathogenesis of acne?

ii. What additional treatments should be considered in this patient?

iii. What drugs or exposures can exacerbate acne or lead to acneiform eruptions?

Answer 15

i. Acne vulgaris is a disorder of the pilosebaceous unit with various clinical presentations, ranging from comedones and inflammatory papules to acne fulminans, a severe form of acne with systemic symptoms such as fever, athralgias, myalgias and malaise. Although typically observed in adolescence, acne can affect all age groups.

The pathogenesis of acne involves the interplay of multiple factors, including genetic predisposition, sebum production, hormonal influences, comedo formation, inflammatory responses and the presence of *Propionibacterium acnes* on the skin. The precise role of genetics is not well understood, but the high concordance rates of acne observed between identical twins and within families support the role of inherited factors such as the number, size and activity of sebaceous glands. Sebum production, which is largely influenced by androgens, contributes to the development of comedonal acne. Comedo formation is the key to the development of acne and results from retained corneocytes accumulating in the follicles, leading to gradual expansion of the comedo and eventual rupture of the comedo wall, releasing its immunogenic and pro-inflammatory contents. *P. acnes* is a Gram-positive rod found within the sebaceous follicles, which contributes to the formation of acne through stimulation of the innate immune system and production of pro-inflammatory mediators such as interleukins that include IL-1, IL-8, IL-12 and tumor necrosis factor-alpha (TNF-α).

ii. Additional treatments that should be considered in this patient with inflammatory acne, in whom numerous topical treatments have failed, include oral antibiotics, oral contraceptives or antiandrogens and oral isotretinoin. Oral tetracycline derivatives (doxycycline, minocycline) or macrolides (erythromycin, azithromycin) are used for their anti-inflammatory properties. In patients who describe a strong association of acne activity with changes in their hormonal levels such as during menstruation, the addition of oral contraceptives can be beneficial. In post-menopausal women, antiandrogens such as spironolactone and flutamide can be used. Oral isotretinoin is used to treat severe, scarring acne or moderate nodulocystic acne that has failed other treatments.

iii. Certain drugs can cause or aggravate acne. These drugs include oral corticosteroids, lithium, anti-epileptic medications such as carbamazepine and phenytoin, azathioprine, cyclosporine and rifampin. Acneiform eruptions can also be seen at sites of prior exposure to therapeutic ionizing radiation.

Epidermal growth factor receptor (EGFR) inhibitors, used to treat solid tumors of the head and neck, lung, colon and breast are another class of drugs that can lead to acneiform eruptions in up to 95% of patients.

CASE 16

Rosacea

QUESTION 16

A 51-year-old woman presents to the Veterans Affairs (VA) dermatology clinic for the evaluation of central facial redness and flushing. She states that this began in her mid-30s and has progressively worsened over time. She notices it more during the summer after sun exposure. She relates associated symptoms of itching, dry skin, occasional burning and warmth with flushing. On examination, there is redness with telangiectasias on the dorsal nose, cheeks and chin (16a).

16a

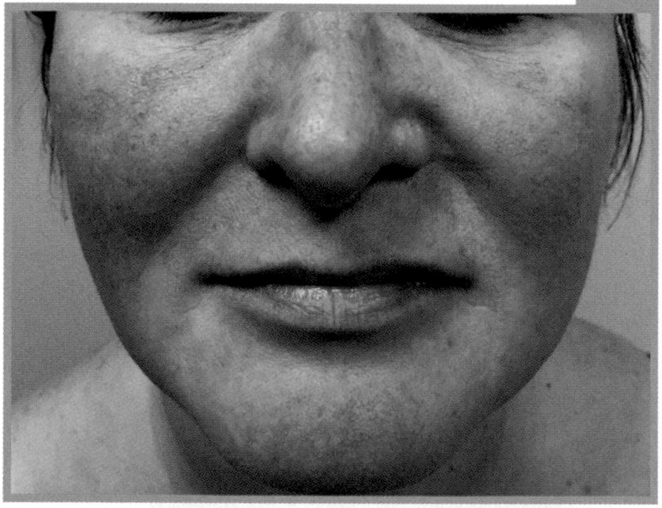

i. What are the four main subtypes of this condition?

ii. What are the main components of the pathogenesis of this condition? What are the microorganisms associated with this condition?

iii. What are the available treatment options?

Answer 16

i. This patient presents with classic features of rosacea, a common chronic inflammatory skin condition. The four main subtypes of rosacea are (1) erythematotelangiectatic, (2) papulopustular, (3) phymatous and (4) ocular rosacea. There are several overlapping features observed across all clinical subtypes of rosacea and patients may present with features of more than one subtype. Erythematotelangiecatic rosacea (ETR) is characterized by persistent central facial erythema and episodes of flushing. The characteristic areas of involvement are the face, ears, neck and upper chest. Papulopustular rosacea (PPR) can have all of the features of ETR, with the addition of transient inflammatory papules, pustules and occasional facial edema in more severe cases. Phymatous rosacea, which is observed more often in men than women, is characterized by thickened, nodular skin affecting areas on the central face, most commonly the nose but occasionally the forehead, cheeks and chin (16b). Ocular rosacea, which can be seen alone or in conjunction with another subtype of rosacea, is defined by the presence of at least one of the following signs or symptoms: dry eyes, itching, burning or stinging, light sensitivity, blurred vision, telangiectasias of the conjunctiva and lid margin, lid or periocular erythema or foreign body sensation.

16b

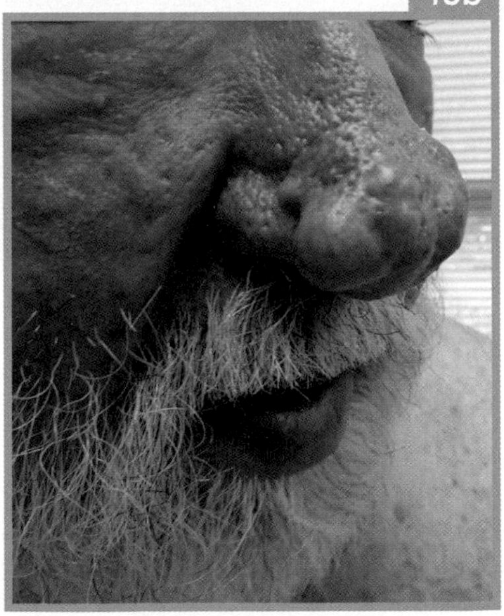

ii. Although the precise pathogenesis is not completely known, a genetic component, dysregulation of the innate immune system, the presence of certain microorganisms, ultraviolet radiation, neurogenic dysregulation and abnormal barrier function may all be involved. The exact role of microorganisms on the skin in the pathogenesis of rosacea is not fully understood, but otherwise healthy individuals with rosacea have a higher density of *Demodex folliculorum* and *Staphylococcus epidermidis* on the skin. In addition, patients with rosacea have a higher prevalence of skin colonization with bacteria that are not typically present on the skin, including *Helicobacter pylori* and *Bacillus oleronius*.

iii. The approach to treatment in patients with rosacea should focus on patient education, skin care and maintenance and medical/procedural interventions. Patients should be aware that there are often specific triggers that can exacerbate rosacea, some of the more common triggers being wind, exercise, spicy foods, physical or psychological stress and hot or cold temperatures. Skin care should incorporate moisturizers to prevent dryness and daily UV protection, as light exposure can exacerbate rosacea.

Topical medications used for mild-to-moderate rosacea include topical sulfacetamide, ivermectin, azelaic acid, metronidazole and brimonidine, an alpha-adrenergic agonist. Topical retinoids, calcineurin inhibitors, macrolides, benzoyl peroxide and permethrin cream are also used off-label. For patients with moderate-to-severe rosacea, tetracycline antibiotics at anti-inflammatory dosing are the mainstay of therapy.

CASE 17

Pseudofolliculitis barbae

QUESTION 17

A 28-year-old African American man presents to the dermatology clinic for the evaluation of recurrent painful razor bumps in the beard distribution. He states that he began developing these lesions after shaving regularly. He has tried numerous aftershave treatments but continues to develop lesions that leave behind dark marks and bumps in the skin. On examination, there are follicular-based hyperpigmented papules along the jawline and anterior neck (17).

17

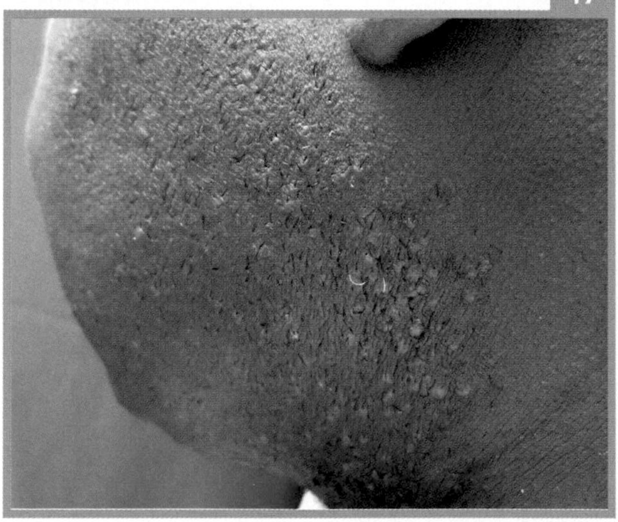

i. What is the diagnosis and etiology of this condition?

ii. What modifications can be made to improve this condition? What treatment options are there?

Answer 17

i. This patient presents with pseudofolliculitis barbae (PFB), an inflammatory disorder that is typically seen in individuals with darkly pigmented skin and tight curly hair. Although it is most commonly seen in African American men in the beard area, women who regularly shave can also develop pseudofolliculitis barbae in the groin and inguinal regions or on the chin in the setting of hirsutism. PFB is thought to occur after shaving due to the growth of a curved hair shaft that penetrates into the skin where the hair exits the follicle. An inflammatory reaction occurs in response to hair keratin penetrating the dermis.

ii. The definitive treatment of pseudofolliculitis barbae is the cessation of shaving. For individuals who plan to continue shaving, shaving methods can be optimized to prevent the development of lesions, such as shaving only in the direction of hair growth, using sharp razors, avoiding shaving over the same areas multiple times, and avoiding very close shaves by pulling the skin taut. Other treatment options include warm compresses with saline or aluminium acetate solutions, low-potency topical steroids, retinoids and clindamycin. Laser hair removal can also be used for definitive treatment, particularly in patients with recalcitrant disease.

CASE 18

Acne keloidalis nuchae

QUESTION 18

A 45-year-old African American man presents to the dermatology clinic for evaluation of painful recurrent bumps on the back of his neck. He began developing painful, pus-filled bumps on the back of his scalp and neck in his early 30s and some have healed with scarring. On examination, there are numerous firm follicular-based papules and keloidal plaques on the occipital scalp with associated areas of alopecia (18).

18

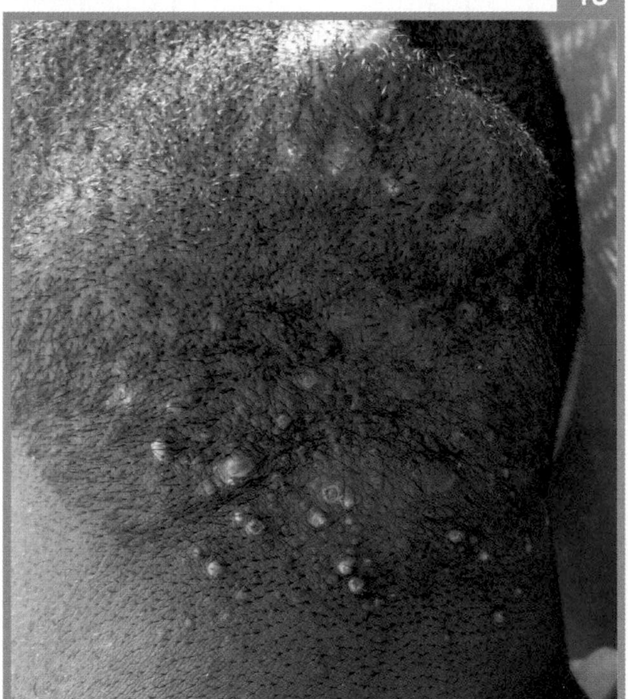

i. What is the diagnosis?

ii. What are the available treatment options?

Answer 18

i. The patient presents with acne keloidalis, also known as acne keloidalis nuchae and folliculitis keloidalis, which is a chronic form of folliculitis and perifolliculitis that is observed almost exclusively in African American men. Acne keloidalis presents as follicular-based papules distributed over the occipital scalp and posterior neck that can be painful and coalesce into keloidal plaques near the posterior hairline. Uncommonly, secondary bacterial infection can occur and lead to drainage. Areas of chronic involvement can lead to associated alopecia.

ii. The first-line of treatment is the prevention of lesions. Patients should be educated regarding avoidance of triggers or factors that can lead to mechanical irritation such as shirt collars, tight-fitting hats or headgear. For the treatment of existing lesions, topical therapy can be initiated with a combination of topical corticosteroids and retinoids. In patients with significant folliculitis, topical or oral antibiotics used for acne vulgaris can also be used with some success. For more extensive disease, intralesional corticosteroids can soften and decrease the appearance of larger, chronic keloidal plaques. Additional therapies for larger plaques and nodules include excision, laser and cryosurgery. Post-operatively, topical imiquimod is a treatment option to prevent recurrence.

CASE 19

Hidradenitis suppurativa

QUESTION 19

A 37-year-old African American woman with a history of depression presents with multiple recurrent abscesses in both axillae and in her inguinal region, many of which have required multiple visits to the emergency department for incision and drainage and multiple repeated courses of oral antibiotics. She states that they began occurring in her 20s and her sister also develops similar lesions. They have now increased in frequency and she is concerned about the scarring and pigmentation changes that the lesions leave behind. On examination, there are subcutaneous hyperpigmented nodules with associated firm scarring tracts, some with white-yellow drainage (19). There are multiple double comedones within the axillae and groin folds.

19

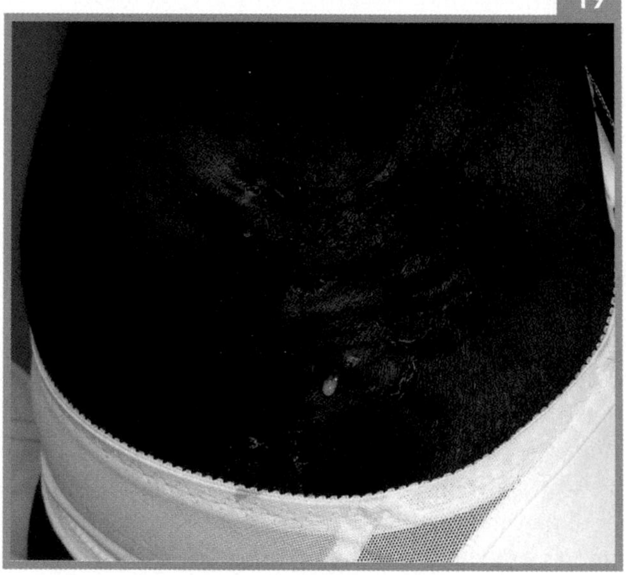

i. What is the diagnosis and how is the severity and extent assessed?

ii. What risk factors are associated with this condition?

iii. In some people, this disease can be part of which clinical syndrome?

iv. What are the treatment options for this patient?

Answer 19

i. The patient presents with hidradenitis suppurativa, also known as acne inversa, which is a disorder involving pilosebaceous units in the intertriginous areas and secondary inflammation of the apocrine glands. It is a chronic condition that has an onset after puberty, is observed in a 3:1 ratio of women to men, and has a higher incidence among African American individuals. It is characterized by the early development of inflammatory nodules and sterile abscesses that develop into sinus tracts and hypertrophic scars. Drainage of serosanguinous material is common.

There are two grading systems, the Hurley staging system and Sartorius score, which are used to assess the severity of disease. The Hurley staging system describes three clinical stages: Stage I consists of a single lesions without sinus tract formation, Stage II consists of more than one lesion or area but with limited sinus tract formation, and Stage III consists of multiple lesions with extensive sinus tracts and scarring. The Sartorius score is a numerical score based on the involved regions, number and type of lesions and presence of sinus tracts. Points are received for the involvement of different body areas, the presence of nodules, fistulas and scars, and the distance between two different lesions (and if they are separated by normal skin).

ii. Risk factors associated with hidradenitis suppurativa include smoking, genetic predisposition, endocrine factors such as obesity, polycystic ovary syndrome, hirsutism, acne and Crohn's disease.

iii. Hidradenitis suppurativa is part of the follicular occlusion tetrad, which includes acne conglobata, dissecting cellulitis, pilonidal sinus and hidradenitis suppurativa.

iv. Depending on the severity of disease, there are multiple treatment options. Lifestyle modifications include weight reduction, smoking cessation, and measures to reduce friction and moisture in intertriginous regions such as loose-fitting clothing, absorbent powders and topical aluminium chloride. Localized therapies include antiseptic soaps, topical antibiotics such as clindamycin, and intralesional steroids. For severe disease, systemic treatments include systemic retinoids, immunosuppressive and anti-inflammatory agents such as prednisone, mycophenolate mofetil, cyclosporine, azathioprine and tumor necrosis factor-alpha (TNF-α) inhibitors such as adalimumab. Surgical excision with grafting is performed for definitive treatment of severe, scarred sinus tracts.

VASCULAR DISORDERS

CASE 20

Leukocytoclastic vasculitis

QUESTION 20

A 50-year-old man presents to the emergency department with a 3-week history of a cutaneous eruption on the trunk and extremities. He states that the lesions began on his chest and abdomen and continued to progress to his arms and legs. Prior to the onset of the rash, he experienced a febrile illness with pharyngitis that was self-limited and resolved after 7 days. On examination, there are scattered petechiae, purpuric patches and plaques with an erythematous border on the trunks and extremities, some palpable and with central hemorrhagic bullae (20).

20

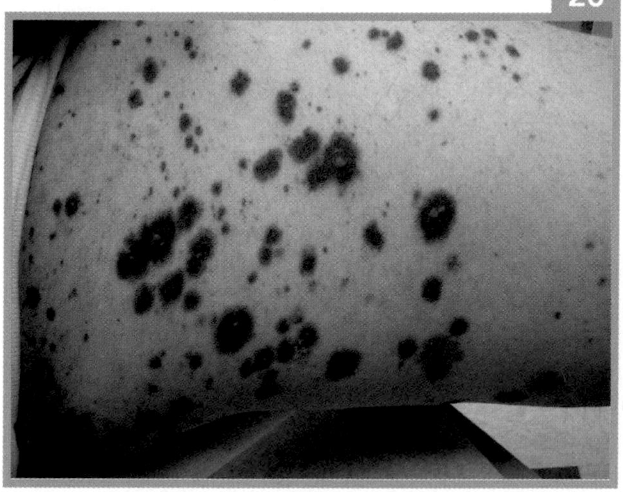

i. What is the most likely cause of these lesions and what are the characteristic histological findings?

ii. What are the common causes of this condition?

iii. What laboratory tests should be performed in the initial work-up of this condition?

Answer 20

i. Based on the history and morphology, the most likely cause of these lesions is a cutaneous small vessel vasculitis process, which is characterized histologically by perivascular infiltrates with neutrophils, karyorrhexis, and erythrocyte extravasation. The pathogenesis of cutaneous small vessel vasculitis involves immune complex deposition within postcapillary venules, which leads to complement activation. Complement activation leads to increased expression of adhesion molecules on the endothelium, mast cell degranulation and neutrophil chemotaxis. These events lead to vascular dilatation and permeability, enhanced immune complex deposition, and the release of proteolytic enzymes and free oxygen radicals by neutrophils, which damage the vessel wall.

Clinically, the lesions of cutaneous small vessel vasculitis tend to occur 7–10 days after exposure to an inciting agent or event. Lesions can range from palpable purpura to erythematous papules and vesicles that favour the dependent areas and areas of trauma. Systemic symptoms are seen in up to 25% of individuals, most often fever, weight loss, myalgias, arthralgias, genitourinary symptoms or gastrointestinal symptoms.

ii. Up to 50% of cases of cutaneous small vessel vasculitis are idiopathic; however, there are many secondary causes of small vessel vasculitis. Other causes of cutaneous small vessel vasculitis include infections, inflammatory disorders, medications and malignancies. Among infectious causes, viral infections (hepatitis C and B) and bacterial infections with beta-hemolytic streptococci, infective endocarditis, *Neisseria meningococcus* and atypical mycobacterial infections are common. Rheumatoid arthritis, systemic lupus erythematosus and Sjogren's syndrome are autoimmune connective tissue diseases that can be associated with cutaneous small vessel vasculitis. Medications that are often implicated include allopurinol, cephalosporins, penicillins, quinolones, sulfonamides, thiazides, non-steroidal anti-inflammatory drugs (NSAIDs) and antithyroid agents. Neoplasms, which only comprise 2%–5% of causes of cutaneous small vessel vasculitis, include plasma cell dyscrasias, myeloproliferative disorders and lymphoproliferative disorders.

iii. In the initial work-up of cutaneous small vessel vasculitis, a comprehensive history of recent illnesses and medication exposures is prudent. Laboratory testing should include a complete blood cell count, comprehensive metabolic panel, and other specific laboratory testing toward other aetiologies of cutaneous small vessel vasculitis such as cultures, hepatitis panel, rheumatoid factor, antinuclear and other autoantibodies, urinalysis, and serum and urine protein electrophoresis.

CASE 21

Levamisole vasculopathy

QUESTION 21

A 37-year-old woman is evaluated by the dermatology consult service in the emergency department, where she presented with a new painful rash on the legs. She reports that the rash began on her legs but quickly spread to her trunk, arms and ears over the past 48 hours. The lesions were initially non-tender but have become intensely tender to palpation. Her past medical history is notable for polysubstance abuse and infective endocarditis. On examination, there are numerous purpuric plaques with irregular, stellate borders. Some of the larger lesions have hemorrhagic bullae in the centre with evidence of necrosis (21).

21

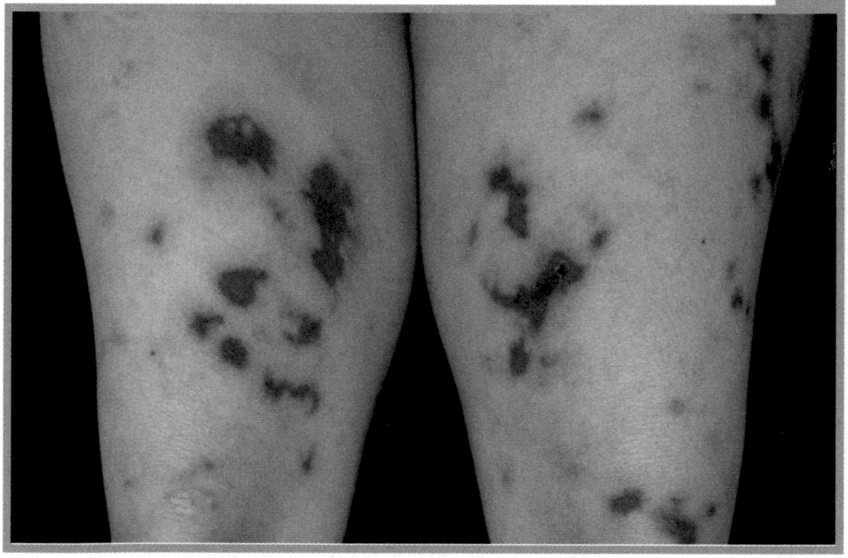

i. What is the diagnosis and causative agent?

ii. What are the other associated findings that can be seen with this condition?

iii. What are the available treatment options?

Answer 21

i. The patient presents with levamisole vasculopathy or retiform purpura due to levamisole-adulterated cocaine. Although levamisole was initially developed as an antihelminthic agent, it has been used more recently for the treatment of rheumatoid arthritis, nephrotic syndrome and colon and breast cancer until it was withdrawn due to adverse effects of agranulocytosis, cutaneous vasculitides and leukoencephalopathy. More recently, it has been used to cut cocaine, detected in >70% of cocaine tested in the United States in 2009. It is thought to increase the euphoric and stimulatory effects of cocaine by forming amphetamine-like metabolites.

Patients who develop levamisole vasculopathy experience an acute onset of a purpuric rash that affects the extremities and trunk and characteristically affects the ears and nose. These lesions often progress to ulceration and necrosis and can lead to significant morbidity due to scarring.

ii. In a review of cases of levamisole vasculopathy, antiphospholipid antibodies and antinuclear cytoplasmic antibodies were detected in 65% and 91% of the cases, respectively.

iii. After withdrawal of the offending agent, skin lesions resolve over 2–3 weeks, but can lead to profound scarring. Serologies normalize within 2–14 months. Treatment involves debridement of wounds and wound care. Eculizumab, a monoclonal antibody that targets the complement protein C5, has been described in a few cases for the treatment of this entity.

CASE 22

Calciphylaxis

QUESTION 22

A 51-year-old woman is evaluated by the dermatology consult service for a new painful purpuric rash on her legs. Her medical history is notable for end-stage renal disease, and she is on hemodialysis three times per week. The rash began on her left calf as a small dark purple area but has continued to spread and become more painful. On examination, there is a purpuric plaque with surrounding erythema and irregular, stellate borders, which is firm and exquisitely tender to gentle palpation (22).

22

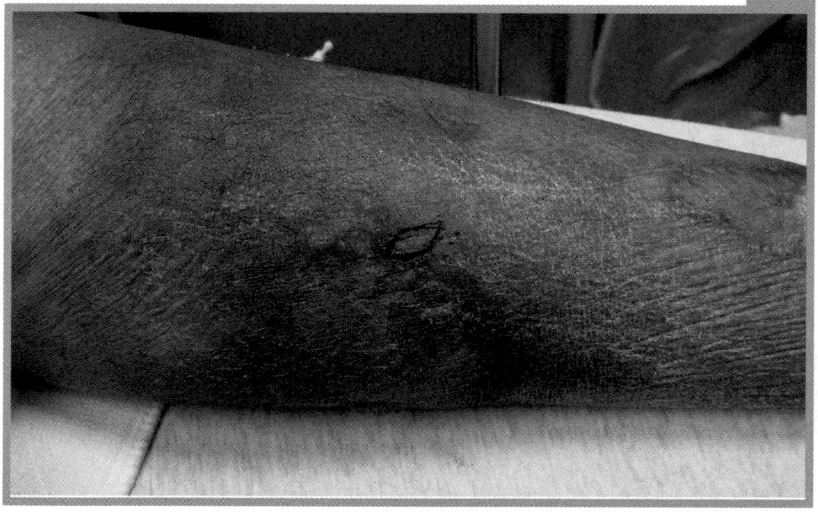

i. What is the most likely diagnosis? What are risk factors for this condition?

ii. What are the characteristic findings on histology?

iii. What are the available treatment options?

Answer 22

i. Calciphylaxis (also known as calcific uremic arteriolopathy), is a phenomenon that occurs in patients with end-stage renal disease and/or hyperparathyroidism, and is characterized by vascular calcification and thrombosis, leading to cutaneous necrosis. It is thought to be caused by elevated levels of serum calcium, phosphate and parathyroid hormone (PTH), often seen in the setting of chronic renal failure. Because of dysfunctional calcium homeostasis, calcium phosphate precipitates in the media of arterioles, leading to vessel injury, intimal fibrosis, thrombosis and cutaneous and soft tissue necrosis. Clinically, calciphylaxis initially presents as an area of fixed livedo reticularis that is firm to the touch and then progresses to become more violaceous, purpuric, bullous and ultimately necrotic. The most common areas of involvement are the legs below the knees (up to 90% of patients), followed by the thighs, buttocks and abdomen.

Up to 4% of patients on hemodialysis and 4% of patients on peritoneal dialysis develop calciphylaxis. Additional risk factors are diabetes mellitus, body mass index (BMI) >30, liver disease, hypoalbuminemia, protein C deficiency and exposure to warfarin or systemic corticosteroids.

ii. Calciphylaxis is a type of metastatic calcification (i.e. it represents calcification in normal tissue) and is associated with elevated serum calcium or phosphate or both. It is characterized by calcified small vessels in the subcutaneous fat with associated necrosis. As vascular calcification is a common finding in patients with end-stage renal disease, this finding alone is not sufficient to confirm the diagnosis of calciphylaxis. Special care must be taken when obtaining a skin biopsy to confirm the diagnosis and excisional biopsies may be required to obtain a specimen that is large and deep enough to demonstrate the diagnostic features.

iii. Calciphylaxis is associated with a mortality rate of 50% at 1 year and 80% at 2 years and is estimated to be even higher in patients with both proximal and distal disease. The most common cause of death is septicemia due to chronic open wounds that are resistant to healing. The treatment of calciphylaxis usually consists of multiple approaches, all targeted towards calcium metabolism. Phosphate binders, low-calcium dialysate and intravenous sodium thiosulfate have been used with varying levels of success. In addition, surgical debridement and hyperbaric oxygen therapy may be helpful for ulcer healing. Parathyroidectomy can be considered in patients with marked elevation of PTH.

CASE 23

Venous malformation

QUESTION 23

A 14-month-old boy presents to the pediatric dermatology clinic as a referral from his pediatrician for the development of multiple painful blue lesions on the leg. The lesions were not present at birth, have become larger over the past several months and seem to cause the child pain. On examination, there are multiple blue-purple subcutaneous nodules that are soft and compressible (23), located on the right thigh and right lower leg.

23

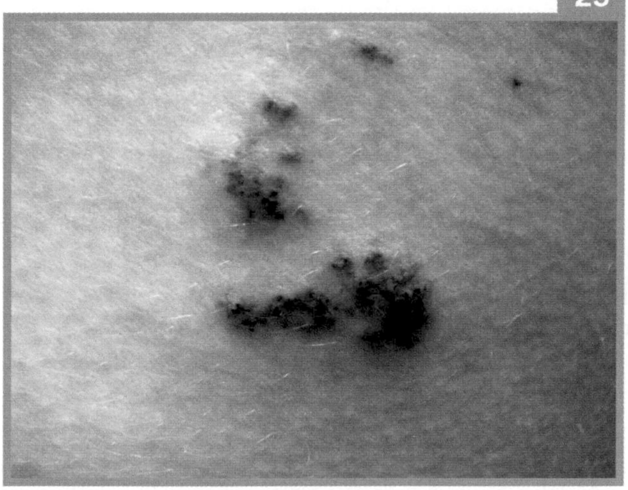

i. What is the most accurate diagnosis?

ii. What type(s) of imaging studies could be performed to confirm the diagnosis?

iii. What syndromes are associated with this finding?

iv. Based on the lesion location, what further assessments and/or considerations should be made?

Answer 23

i. The patient presents with venous malformations (VMs), which can be diagnosed clinically by the blue hue and soft compressible nature of the lesions. These lesions can be focal, segmental or widespread. Depending on the location, VMs can lead to cosmetic and functional problems.

ii. Venous malformations can be best characterized on T2-weighted magnetic resonance imaging (MRI). Other imaging that can be done include ultrasound and computed tomography (CT) imaging with contrast.

iii. Familial cutaneous and mucosal venous malformation is an autosomal dominant condition caused by a sporadic mutation in the *TEK* gene found on chromosome 9. It is characterized by multiple VMs on the skin, oral mucosa and muscles and less commonly in the viscera such as the gastrointestinal (GI) tract, lungs, brain and heart. Glomuvenous malformation is an autosomal dominant syndrome due to mutation in the glomulin gene located on chromosome 1. It is characterized by solitary lesions or widespread blue–purple nodules that present at birth or appear in childhood and worsen over time. VMs are usually seen on the skin and occasionally mucosa or superficial muscle and rarely involve the joints or viscera. Blue rubber bleb nevus syndrome (BRBNS) is a sporadic disease with widespread blue papules and nodules that can involve the GI tract and result in bleeding and iron deficiency anemia, but typically does not have other visceral involvement. No specific mutations have been identified in this syndrome.

iv. Imaging can be performed to confirm the diagnosis as well as evaluate the extent and depth of involvement. VMs located on the head and neck areas can be associated with various complications. On the head, underlying bony defects or brain developmental venous anomalies may occur. On the eye, VMs can cause broadened bones or enophthalmos. VMs on the cheeks or tongue can lead to abnormal jaw growth, shift of the dental midline and bite deformity while lip involvement can cause labial incompetence. On the pharynx, potential complications include sleep apnea and pharyngeal obstruction. On the trunk, evaluation for underlying visceral involvement such as the pleura, intestines, liver or spleen is appropriate. VMs located on the limbs can be associated with undergrowth (more often than overgrowth) and when overlying a joint, they can lead to joint effusion, hemarthrosis or contracture. Underlying bone issues can be seen such as osteoporosis, lytic lesions, bony distortion or pathological fractures. Patients with extensive VMs should also be evaluated for localized intravascular coagulopathy with routine laboratory work-up including D-dimer, platelet count, prothrombin time and partial thromboplastin time.

RHEUMATOLOGIC DERMATOLOGY

CASE 24

Dermatomyositis

QUESTION 24

A 51-year-old woman presents to the dermatology clinic with a pruritic rash on her face and upper chest, present for 9 months. She reports that the rash is particularly prominent in the summer months when exposed to the sun and she has tried multiple treatments including sunscreen and topical steroids. She has also undergone patch testing and removed potential allergens from her daily cleansers, moisturizers and cosmetic products. She complains of general fatigue and weakness in her arms and legs. She has a medical history significant for hypertension, hyperlipidemia and early-onset arthritis. On examination, there is erythema and edema of the central face and eyelids (24a) and on the hands, there are telangiectasias on the nail folds (24b).

24a

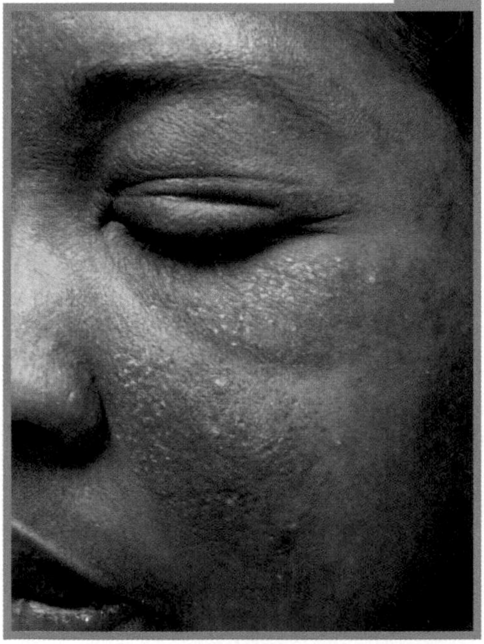

24b

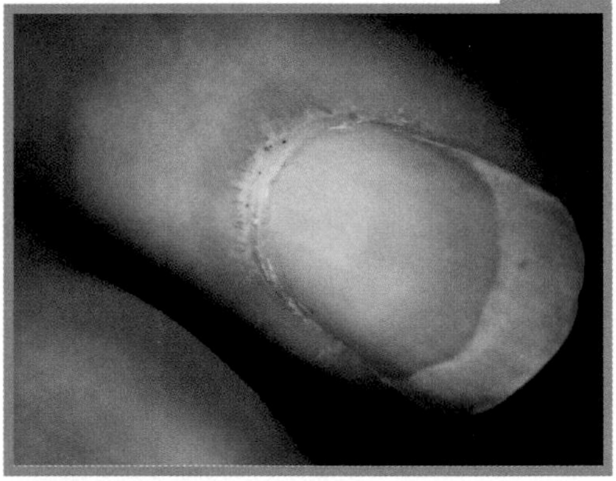

i. What is the diagnosis and what systemic symptoms are associated with this disease?

ii. What are the other laboratory findings that support this diagnosis?

iii. What are the characteristic features of this disease on histopathological exam?

iv. What other special considerations should the clinician be aware of in the context of this disease?

Answer 24

i. This patient has dermatomyositis (DM), a rare autoimmune connective tissue disease that falls within the category of inflammatory dermatomyopathies. It occurs more often in women in the age of 50–70 years. The age distribution of dermatomyositis is bimodal, as there is a juvenile variant that presents in children between the ages of 7 and 12 years. The hallmark cutaneous finding in DM is violaceous poikiloderma with dyspigmentation, telangiectasias and epidermal atrophy. Poikiloderma is often photodistributed, affecting the face and upper chest while sparing the nasolabial fold and submental neck. Eyelid edema and violaceous coloring around the eye (known as the heliotrope sign) are characteristic. Nail fold changes of DM include 'ragged' cuticles or cuticular dystrophy and nail fold telangiectasias (24b). Violaceous lichenified papules on the knuckles are known as Gottron's papules, while violaceous plaques on the elbows and/or knees are known as Gottron's sign. Calcinosis cutis, the deposition of calcium in the skin, is seen more commonly in the juvenile form.

Adult-onset DM can be classified as classic, classic with malignancy, classic as part of an overlapping connective tissue disorder, amyopathic and hypomyopathic. Patients often present with malaise and low energy. The myopathy of DM symmetrically affects the proximal muscle groups, particularly the triceps and quadriceps.

ii. Elevation in serum levels of muscle enzymes such as creatinine kinase and aldolase support the diagnosis. Other abnormal lab values that may be seen include elevated aspartate and alanine transaminases and lactate dehydrogenase, released from damaged muscle. Serum antinuclear autoantibodies are often present in adult and juvenile DM, as well as other myositis-specific autoantibodies. In a subset of patients (usually with overlap syndromes), antisynthetase antibodies are present. The term 'antisynthetase syndrome' is used to describe patients with antisynthetase antibodies, fever, erosive polyarthritis, 'mechanic's hands', Raynaud's phenomenon and interstitial lung disease.

iii. Histopathology from skin biopsies in dermatomyositis can be subtle and include epidermal atrophy with vacuolar keratinocyte degeneration, interstitial mucin deposition in the dermis and a sparse lymphocytic infiltrate. Muscle biopsies, preferably taken from the triceps muscle, demonstrate type II muscle fiber atrophy, necrosis, regeneration and hypertrophy with perifascicular and perivascular lymphocytes.

iv. Malignancies have been associated with dermatomyositis with reported frequency ranging from 10% to 50%. Genitourinary and colon cancers have been reported most often, followed by lymphomas, breast, lung, gastric and pancreatic cancers. There appears to be an increased risk of malignancy in patients with amyopathic DM. Vigilance and age-appropriate cancer screening are of paramount importance in patients with dermatomyositis, particularly within the first 2–5 years after diagnosis.

CASE 25

Discoid lupus erythematosus

QUESTION 25

A 49-year-old African American woman presents to the dermatology clinic with an area of hypopigmentation on the left ear that has become progressively painful. She does not have any other areas of involvement and denies a history of trauma to the area. She also notes a history of patchy hair loss and arthritis of her ankles. Recent urine studies show incidental finding of proteinuria. In her family history, her mother suffers from hypertension, cardiovascular disease and end-stage renal disease. On examination, there is a hypopigmented patch on the left ear with evidence of scaling, central atrophy and mild hyperpigmentation at the periphery (25).

25

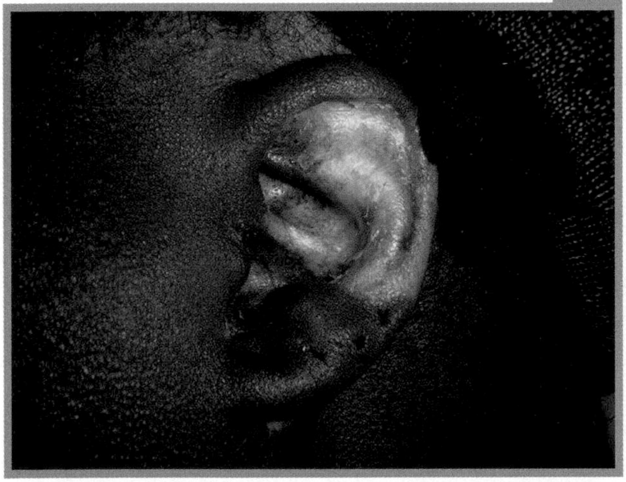

i. What is the most likely diagnosis?

ii. What are other clinical and laboratory findings that support this diagnosis?

iii. What are the characteristic features of this disease on histopathological exam?

iv. What are the signs of systemic involvement?

Answer 25

i. Based on this patient's clinical history and findings, the most likely diagnosis is discoid lupus erythematosus (DLE), one of the most common cutaneous manifestations of lupus erythematosus and a clinical variant of chronic cutaneous lupus erythematosus. Lesions of DLE favor the head and neck and can demonstrate erythema, scaling, atrophy and dyspigmentation. Discoid lesions often remain over prolonged periods and can lead to permanent scarring. Involvement of the scalp can result in scarring alopecia, although there is also an increased incidence of alopecia areata among patients with lupus erythematosus.

Although systemic lupus erythematosus (SLE) is more often associated with the acute form of cutaneous lupus erythematosus, it can also occur with DLE. Between 1% and 5% of patients with DLE may develop SLE and an estimated 25% of patients with SLE may develop typical discoid lesions at some point during the course of the disease. Additional history provided in this vignette, indicates that this patient likely has SLE with joint and renal involvement.

ii. Other non-specific cutaneous findings that support the diagnosis of lupus erythematosus include vascular lesions such as livedo reticularis, palmar erythema, Raynaud's phenomenon, periungual telangiectasias, purpura, urticarial papules or ulcerations, as well as alopecia, sclerodactyly, calcinosis cutis and rheumatoid nodules. These findings are not specific to lupus and can be seen in other connective tissue disorders or in overlap syndromes with SLE. Laboratory values that may assist in making the diagnosis of SLE include antinuclear antibody, anti-double stranded DNA antibody, urinalysis, erythrocyte sedimentation rate and complement levels (C3, C4).

iii. Characteristic histological findings of DLE include vacuolar alteration of the basilar layer of the epidermis, thickening of the basement membrane zone, follicular plugging and dermal and periadnexal lymphocytic infiltrates.

iv. Lupus erythematosus can potentially affect multiple organ systems in addition to the skin, including the joints, pulmonary, cardiac, renal, hematologic and central nervous systems. This can manifest as non-erosive arthritis of peripheral joints, pleuritis or pericarditis, proteinuria or cellular casts, hemolytic anemia, leukopenia, lymphopenia, thrombocytopenia, seizures or psychosis.

CASE 26

Scleroderma

QUESTION 26

A 38-year-old woman presents with a history of edema in her hands, pain and stiffness in her fingers with colour changes during the winter. She complains of painful ulcerations on the digital pulp of her fingertips that heal with scars. She also notes areas of asymptomatic dilated blood vessels on her lips that she finds unsightly. On examination, there are pitted scars on the tips of the fingers with some associated atrophy (26).

26

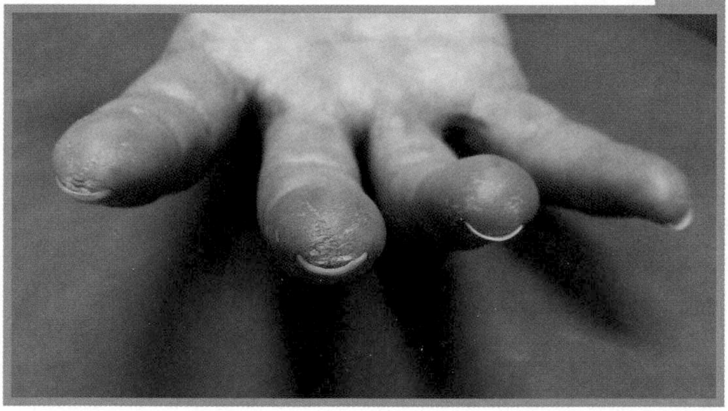

i. Based on this patient's clinical presentation, what is the most likely diagnosis?

ii. What basic laboratory studies can be performed to confirm the diagnosis and what additional screening tests can be performed?

Answer 26

i. This patient is presenting with systemic sclerosis (SSc), also known as scleroderma and progressive systemic sclerosis, which is an autoimmune connective tissue disease that affects the skin, blood vessels and visceral organs. There are two major clinical subtypes of systemic sclerosis: limited and diffuse. In the limited subtype of systemic sclerosis, fibrotic changes in the skin are limited to the fingers, hands and face. Classic cutaneous features involving the hands include pitting edema of the digits, a taut shiny appearance of the skin and flexion contractures and ulcers. In the face, contractures can lead to a beaked nose and microstomia. Matted or squared off telangiectasias are other common skin findings, seen on the face, lips and palms of patients with limited SSc. CREST syndrome is a variant of limited SSc and is an acronym for the clinical features of this entity, which include *c*alcinosis, *R*aynaud's phenomenon, *e*sophageal involvement, *s*clerodactyly and *t*elangiectasias. In this patient, the most likely diagnosis is limited SSc, given the involvement of the fingers and face.

Diffuse SSc occurs when the skin disease involves distal and proximal portions of the extremities, the trunk and the face. Internal organ involvement can be seen with both subtypes, but the diffuse variant is typically associated with visceral involvement within the first 5 years of disease onset and is associated with a worse prognosis. The most common organ systems involved in SSc are the gastrointestinal tract, lung, heart and kidneys.

The diagnosis of systemic sclerosis can be made based on the classification scheme of the American College of Rheumatology, which includes one major criterion: symmetric cutaneous sclerosis proximal to the metacarpophalangeal or metatarsophalangeal joints; or ≥2 minor criteria, which include: sclerodactyly, digital pitted scars or loss of substance of finger pads and bibasilar pulmonary fibrosis.

ii. The presence of antinuclear autoantibodies has been reported in 80%–98% of the SSc cases. Classically, the autoantibodies detected are anti-centromere and anti-topoisomerase I in up to 50%–60% of patients with SSc. Further diagnostic tests to appropriately define the stage of patients with systemic sclerosis include esophageal manometry and pH-metry, lung vital capacity and diffusing capacity for carbon monoxide, intrarenal duplex Doppler sonography, echocardiography and skin plicometry.

CASE 27

Morphea

QUESTION 27

A 63-year-old woman presents to the dermatology clinic with an enlarging scar-like area behind her ear. The area has grown progressively over 2 years and has become increasingly tight, uncomfortable and pruritic. The area is hard, raised and erythematous with central scarring and atrophy (27). Her medical history is significant only for hypertension and osteoarthritis.

27

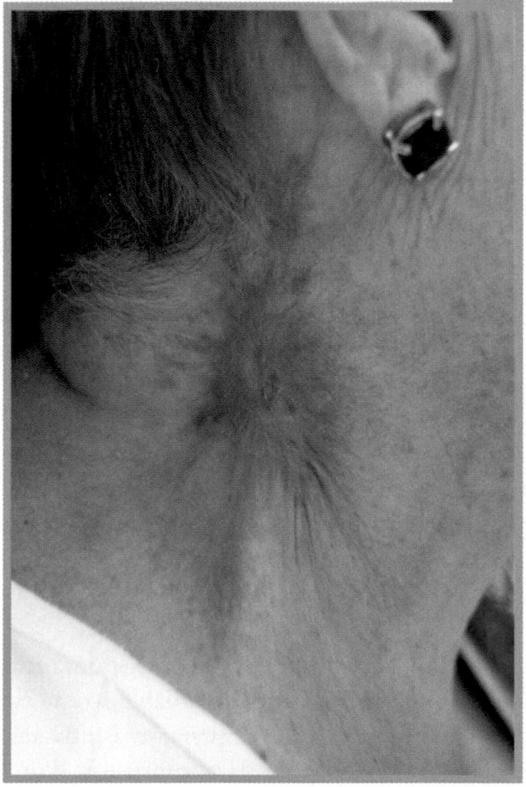

i. What is the most likely diagnosis?

ii. What are the potential complications of this disease?

iii. What are the treatment options?

Answer 27

i. Based on this patient's clinical presentation, the most likely diagnosis is morphea, an inflammatory disease in the dermis and subcutaneous structures. The main variants include plaque-type, linear and generalized morphea.

The most common variant is plaque-type morphea, which is characterized by the development of erythematous to violaceous plaques that expand radially over several years with central sclerosis. The lesions are usually asymptomatic, but more advanced lesions can cause discomfort and skin tightness owing to the progressive scarring and induration of the skin. Although these lesions usually resolve spontaneously over a course of years, they can lead to permanent atrophy and changes in pigmentation. Relapsing disease is uncommon in plaque-type morphea.

Linear morphea is a clinical variant that often presents as a linear, inflammatory streak or an initial plaque-type lesion that extends longitudinally to form a scar band. One specific type of linear morphea is known as morphea *en coup de sabre,* which refers to linear morphea of the forehead and scalp. Generalized morphea is a rare clinical variant that occurs when multiple plaque-type lesions arise at once and become confluent to involve almost all of the total body skin surface area.

ii. Morphea is a disease process that is localized to the skin and does not involve internal organs. However, in the linear morphea variant, the underlying fascia, muscle and bone can be involved, leading to impairment of mobility. High-risk areas are those overlying the joints, which can lead to joint immobility. Morphea *en coup de sabre* can also involve underlying muscles and osseous structures and rarely progress to involve the eye, meninges, or brain. In the generalized form, the diffuse sclerosis can lead to vasoconstriction leading to symptoms such as difficulty breathing as a result of impaired thorax mobility and inflammation of the intercostal muscles.

iii. Although typical plaque-type morphea regresses spontaneously over several years, there are several treatment options available to expedite resolution. Phototherapy with UVA1 or bath PUVA therapy is efficacious in providing faster clinical improvement and longer periods of remission. For systemic treatments, immunosuppression with oral corticosteroids or methotrexate can be helpful during the acute inflammatory stages. There is some evidence supporting the efficacy of oral vitamin A derivatives such as etretinate or acitretin. Topical therapy plays a smaller role in the treatment of morphea. High-potency topical steroids, calcineurin inhibitors and vitamin D derivatives may help reduce local inflammation in acute lesions, but overall are ineffective by themselves in resolving the lesions.

CASE 28

En coup de sabre

QUESTION 28

A 61-year-old woman presents to the dermatology clinic for evaluation of a linear scar down her forehead. She states that it has been present for about 2 months and began as a slightly depressed scar with surrounding hair loss at her frontal hairline that has progressed down to the glabellar region. She also reports more frequent headaches over the last month, for which she is taking acetaminophen. Her past medical history is significant for hypothyroidism and type II diabetes mellitus. On examination, there is an erythematous, linear depression from the frontoparietal scalp to the glabella with prominent veins and associated alopecia (28). On review of systems, she reports headaches and denies seizures, vision change or weight loss.

28

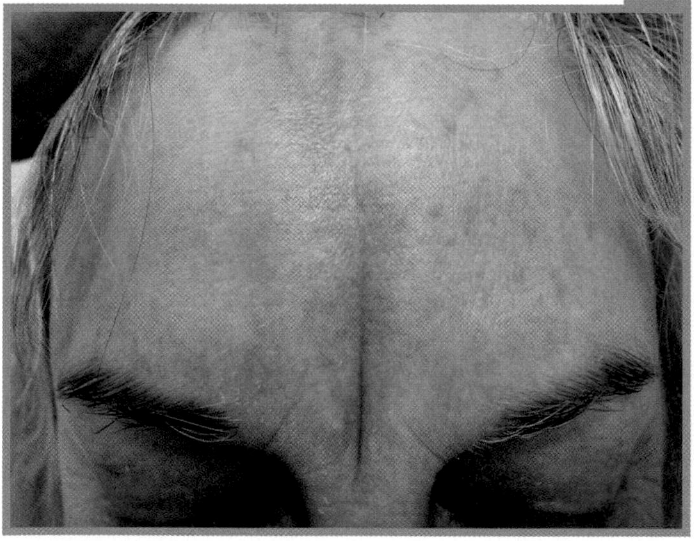

i. What is the most likely diagnosis?

ii. What other concerns are associated with this cutaneous finding?

iii. What are some of the laboratory findings that support this diagnosis?

Answer 28

i. This patient presents with *en coup de sabre* morphea, a subtype of linear morphea that involves the forehead and scalp. Linear morphea can be seen in children and adults, but peak incidence is observed around the fifth decade of life. It is seen more commonly in light-skinned individuals and it is more prevalent in women than men in a 2.6:1 ratio. There may be an increased prevalence of autoimmune disorders associated with linear morphea, but family history is uncommon.

The hallmark finding in this disease is an atrophic linear lesion in the frontoparietal area that usually affects the skin and subcutaneous tissue, although there can be underlying muscle, cartilage and bone involvement. The lesions are typically paramedian and associated alopecia is a common finding.

ii. In *en coup de sabre* morphea, underlying muscle, cartilage and bone lesions can occur. In these cases, there are additional concerns for associated neurologic abnormalities. Nervous system involvement includes headache, epilepsy, focal neurologic deficits, movement disorders and neuropsychiatric symptoms such as behavioural changes or intellectual deterioration.

Parry–Romberg syndrome is a severe variant of linear morphea that affects the face. It is characterized by hemifacial atrophy that can affect the entire distribution of the trigeminal nerve.

iii. The diagnosis of *en coup de sabre* is primarily a clinical diagnosis. Although there are no specific diagnostic laboratory tests, up to 50% of patients with linear morphea may have a positive antinuclear antibody and anti-single-stranded-DNA antibody test.

PANNICULITIS AND PERFORATING DISEASES

CASE 29

Erythema nodosum

QUESTION 29

A 40-year-old woman presents to the dermatology clinic with a painful rash on the lower legs. The rash appeared suddenly on her bilateral legs with firm, painful nodules underneath the skin and seemed to spread within 1 week. Her medical history is notable for hypertension, poorly controlled Crohn's disease and fibromyalgia. On physical examination, there are numerous red-brown subcutaneous nodules that are painful to the touch on the patient's anterior lower legs (29). A biopsy is performed and demonstrates a septal panniculitis with lymphocytes and scattered neutrophils.

29

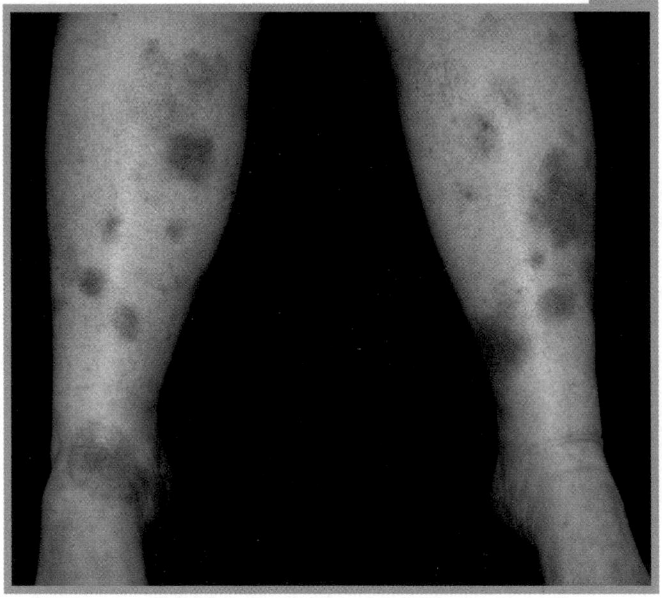

i. What is the diagnosis?

ii. What are the common causes of this condition?

iii. What is the prognosis and treatment?

Answer 29

i. This patient presents with erythema nodosum (EN), which is a form of panniculitis that is considered to be a delayed hypersensitivity reaction. It can occur at any age and is seen equally across different sex and races. Erythema nodosum characteristically presents as painful erythematous subcutaneous nodules, most often located symmetrically on the anterior shins, thighs and forearms. Occasionally, systemic symptoms can be associated with EN, including arthritis, arthralgia, fever and malaise.

ii. Erythema nodosum is often observed in the setting of various systemic diseases, although the largest proportion of cases (up to 50%) is categorized as idiopathic. Infections are common causes of EN, most commonly streptococcal infections and less often, bacterial gastroenteritis and viral upper respiratory tract infections. Other causes of EN include drugs such as estrogens and oral contraceptives, penicillin and biologic agents, sarcoidosis and inflammatory bowel disease, with a stronger association observed between EN and Crohn's disease than with ulcerative colitis. Less common causes of EN include *Chlamydia trachomatis* infections, *Mycoplasma pneumonia* infections, tuberculosis, hepatitis B, Sweet's syndrome and pregnancy.

In the setting of Crohn's disease, EN can be seen prior to or contemporaneously with a flare. The presence of EN is considered as a prognostic factor in some instances; EN is associated with a more benign and self-limited form of sarcoidosis.

iii. The treatment of uncomplicated, mild EN consists of bed rest, nonsteroidal anti-inflammatory drugs (NSAIDs) and potassium iodide. For more severe cases, colchicine, prednisone, dapsone and hydroxychloroquine have been used with success in a small series of patients. Treatment of the underlying condition is an important component of the management of erythema nodosum.

CASE 30

Lipodermatosclerosis

QUESTION 30

A 54-year-old woman presents to the dermatology clinic as a referral from her primary care physician for evaluation of painful induration and hardening of the skin on her lower legs bilaterally. She has a medical history notable for obesity, coronary artery disease, type II diabetes mellitus, peripheral neuropathy and chronic venous insufficiency. She has been treated with two courses of systemic antibiotics for cellulitis of the lower legs but notes no improvement in her symptoms. On examination, there is localized, well-demarcated induration with some sclerotic changes and associated hyperpigmentation affecting the distal medial leg above the malleolus (30).

30

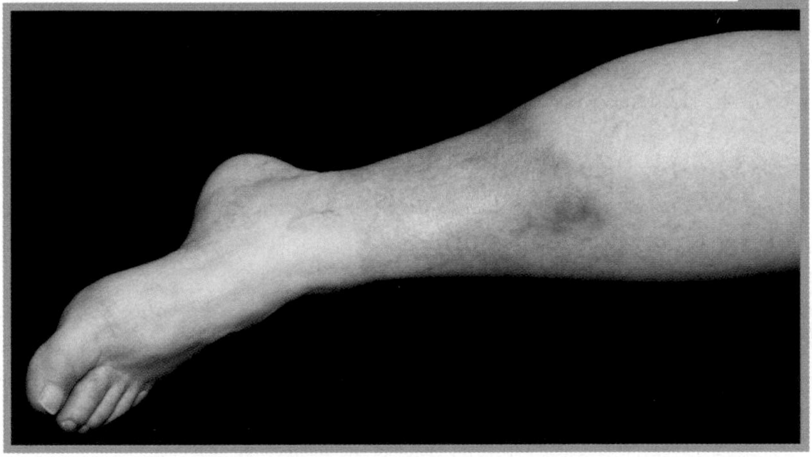

i. What is the diagnosis? What factors contribute to the pathogenesis of this disorder?

ii. What are the characteristic features seen on histopathologic examination?

iii. What is the mainstay of treatment?

Answer 30

i. This patient presents with lipodermatosclerosis, also known as sclerosing panniculitis. It is usually observed in the setting of chronic venous insufficiency. The pathogenesis is thought to occur as a result of venous hypertension, which leads to increased capillary permeability and leakage of fibrinogen. The presence of fibrinogen results in the formation of fibrin cuffs around vessels, which hinders oxygen exchange and leads to tissue anoxia. Additional factors that contribute to the pathogenesis of lipodermatosclerosis include the abnormal regulation of angiogenesis (increased expression of vascular endothelial growth factor receptor 1 and of angiopoietin-2), protein C and S deficiencies and obesity.

In the acute phase, lipodermatosclerosis can resemble cellulitis. However, the failure to improve with antibiotics and surrounding stasis changes can help accurately identify the diagnosis. In the chronic phase, sclerosis in the dermis and subcutis lead to well-demarcated induration that imparts an 'inverted wine bottle' appearance to the affected leg(s).

ii. In acute lipodermatosclerosis, there are inflammatory infiltrates in the septa around fat lobules, evidence of capillary congestion and thrombosis and hemosiderin deposition. In chronic lesions, the inflammatory component is reduced and there is marked septal sclerosis and lipomembranous changes, which consists of thickened membranes with cyst formation in papillary configurations. Although lipomembranous changes are characteristic of lipodermatosclerosis, they can also be observed in panniculitis seen in the setting of lupus and dermatomyositis, erythema nodosum and diabetic dermopathy.

iii. The mainstays of therapy for lipodermatosclerosis are leg elevation and compression therapy. Anabolic steroids such as danazol and oxandrolone enhance fibrinolysis and can help to reduce the pain and induration of the skin.

CASE 31

Elastosis perforans serpiginosa

QUESTION 31

A 14-year-old boy presents to the dermatology clinic for evaluation of a spreading rash on the neck and arms. He was seen by his pediatrician and was initially diagnosed with tinea corporis and prescribed topical antifungal medications. However, he noted no improvement and his parents noticed spreading of the lesions. He denies any symptoms including pruritus. His medical history is notable for Ehlers–Danlos syndrome. On physical examination, there are erythematous hyperkeratotic papules arranged in a polycyclic and serpiginous pattern on the posterior neck and left forearm, with central clearing (31a, b).

31a

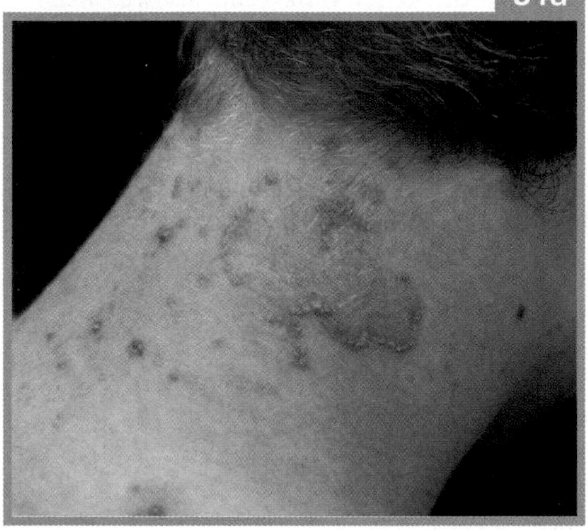

31b

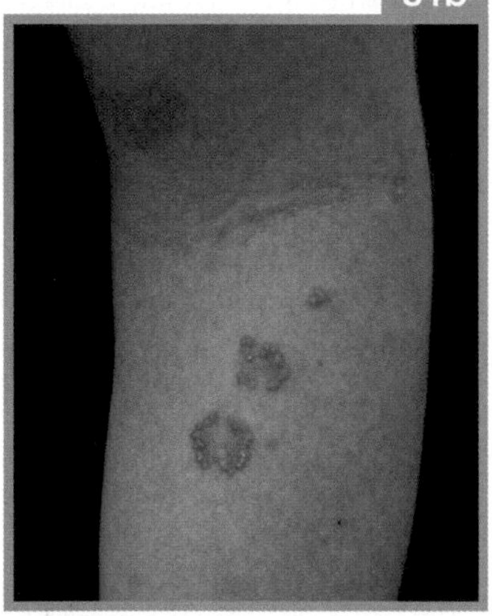

i. What is the diagnosis and what are the treatment options?

ii. What are the characteristic features on histopathologic examination?

iii. What syndromes are associated with this condition?

Answer 31

i. The patient's lesions are consistent with elastosis perforans serpiginosa (EPS), a perforating disorder of the skin. In this condition, abnormal elastic fibres pass through the papillary dermis upwards to the epidermis. Clinically, it is characterized by keratotic papules arranged in an annular or polycyclic pattern that favour the neck, arms and flexures. Although it can occasionally be mildly pruritic, EPS is often asymptomatic and can be monitored.

Treatment of EPS can be challenging. Although it can spontaneously resolve over the course of years without complications, it can also be treated with cryotherapy, excision, pulsed dye laser or cellophane tape stripping.

ii. Histopathologically, EPS will demonstrate abnormal, thickened elastic fibres in the dermis and extruding through an acanthotic epidermis. Elastic tissue stains can be performed, which will highlight the thickened bulky appearance of the elastic tissue.

iii. Up to 40% of cases of EPS are observed within the setting of other genetic disorders including Ehlers–Danlos syndrome, Down syndrome, Marfan syndrome, Rothmund–Thomson syndrome, pseudoxanthoma elasticum and osteogenesis imperfecta. EPS can also be seen in association with renal failure as well as penicillamine use.

NEUTROPHILIC AND GRANULOMATOUS DERMATOSES

CASE 32

Sweet's syndrome

QUESTION 32

A 64-year-old Caucasian woman is evaluated by the inpatient dermatology consult service after being admitted to the hospital for an acute onset of high fever and a rash on the dorsal hands, neck and face. Two weeks prior to her presentation, the patient noticed easy bruising, nosebleeds and fatigue. A review of systems is positive for fever, arthralgia and sensitivity to light. On examination, the surrounding skin on the dorsum of the hands is erythematous and tender to touch. There are multiple edematous hemorrhagic bullae, which have developed over the last 24 hours of her hospital admission (32). A CBC reveals a white cell count of 37,000 cells per microlitre with 10% blasts. A skin biopsy is performed and histopathologic examination demonstrates superficial papillary edema along with numerous polymorphonuclear leukocytes, some of which exhibit karyorrhexis, within the papillary and mid-dermis.

32

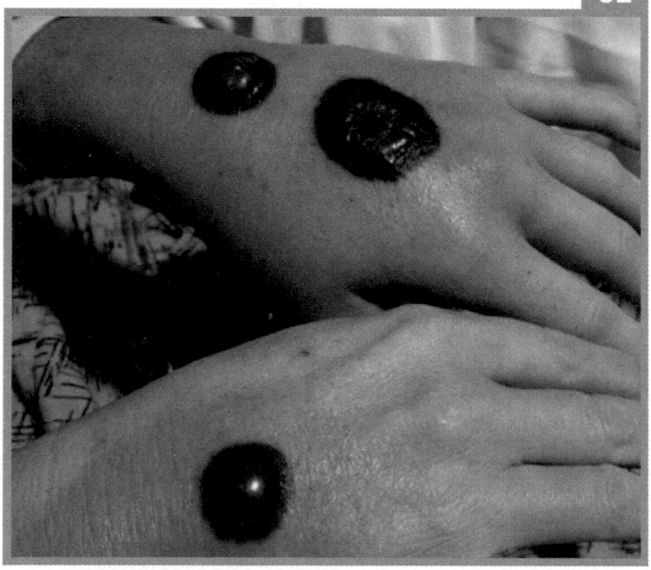

i. What is the most likely diagnosis based on the clinical and pathologic findings?

ii. What is the most likely underlying condition?

iii. What are the diagnostic criteria for this condition?

iv. What is the first-line treatment for the cutaneous disease?

Answer 32

i. This patient presents with Sweet's syndrome, also known as acute febrile neutrophilic dermatosis. This is an uncommon condition typically seen in adults, and with a female-to-male predominance (4:1). The clinical features of Sweet's syndrome include initially tender erythematous papules or plaques that favour the head, neck and upper extremities. They are often characterized by pronounced edema that may produce a pseudovesicular or pseudopustular appearance. These lesions can develop further into vesicles, bullae or pustules that can be hemorrhagic.

On histopathologic examination, Sweet's syndrome demonstrates characteristic nodular and perivascular neutrophilic infiltrates without evidence of vasculitis throughout the dermis. In the epidermis, there can be significant epidermal spongiosis and papillary edema.

ii. Up to 20% of patients with Sweet's syndrome have internal malignancies. Given this patient's cutaneous findings, symptoms and laboratory findings, the most likely underlying condition is acute myelogenous leukemia (AML). The vesiculobullous variant is most frequently associated with AML, and can often mimic superficial pyoderma gangrenosum due to the development of ulcerations. Sweet's syndrome can also be associated with other inflammatory and autoimmune disorders such as inflammatory bowel disease, and can be drug-induced, pregnancy-related, or post-infectious.

iii. For the diagnosis of Sweet's syndrome there are two major criteria and four minor criteria. Both major criteria and at least two minor criteria are needed for the diagnosis.

Diagnostic criteria for Sweet's syndrome	
Major criteria	Minor criteria
1. Abrupt onset of typical cutaneous lesions 2. Histopathology consistent with Sweet's syndrome	1. Presence of fever, constitutional signs and symptoms 2. Leukocytosis 3. Response to systemic corticosteroids 4. Association with known preceding infection or vaccinations, association with malignancy or inflammatory disorder, association with drug exposure or pregnancy

iv. The first-line treatment for Sweet's syndrome is systemic prednisone, usually at a dose of 0.5–1.0 mg/kg/day for 4–6 weeks.

CASE 33

Pyoderma gangrenosum

QUESTION 33

A 57-year-old Caucasian man with a history of Crohn's disease presents to the gastroenterology clinic with a peristomal ulceration. The ulcer is intensely tender and has grown larger and more painful within the last 3 weeks. He was referred to the dermatology clinic, where he presented with a bright red exophytic nodule on the abdomen with an adjacent gun-metal grey ulcerated plaque (33). An incisional punch biopsy was performed at the edge of the ulceration and histopathologic examination revealed ulceration with a neutrophilic inflammatory infiltrate without granulomatous inflammation. The patient's past medical history is notable for a subtotal colectomy for medically refractory Crohn's disease.

33

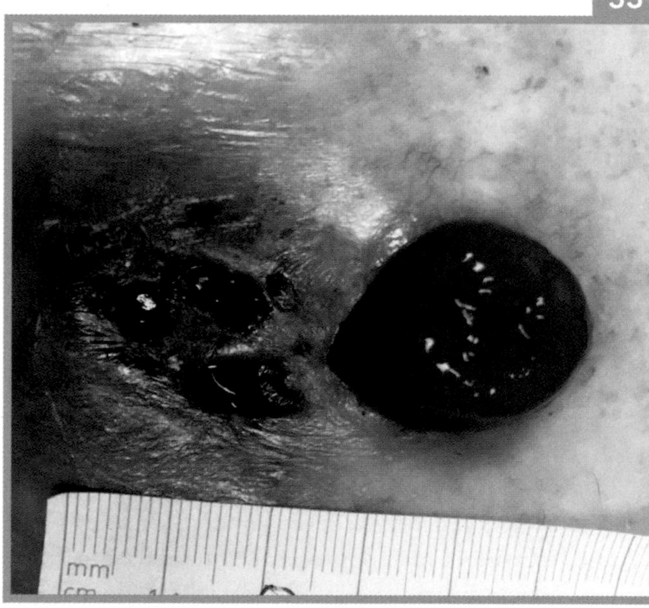

i. What is the most likely diagnosis?

ii. What are the different clinical variants of this disease?

iii. What are the treatment options?

Answer 33

i. The most likely diagnosis is pyoderma gangrenosum (PG), a chronic ulcerative neutrophilic dermatosis. Up to 50% of patients with PG have an associated systemic disease, the most common of which include inflammatory bowel disease (IBD), polyarthritis or hematologic disorders such as immunoglobulin A (IgA) monoclonal gammopathy, acute myelogenous leukemia and myelodysplasia. Although typically observed in adults, approximately 4% of cases are seen in infants and children. The pathogenesis of PG is not completely understood, but the current understanding is that PG develops due to an underlying immunologic abnormality. Lesions of PG demonstrate pathergy, which is the development and/or worsening of skin lesions in response to minor trauma.

In the setting of IBD that requires operative management with bowel resection, peristomal PG can be observed. Studies on the risk factors for developing peristomal PG have demonstrated that female gender, the presence of other concurrent autoimmune disorders and a high body mass index may be contributing factors.

ii. The classic presentation of PG is an ulcer that begins as a tender erythematous papule. Vesiculobullous PG, also known as atypical or bullous PG, presents as vesicles and bullae that tend to favour the face and dorsal hands and arms, which often overlaps in appearance with bullous Sweet's syndrome. This variant is seen most commonly in the setting of hematologic disorders. The pustular variant of PG presents as multiple pustules that typically regress but can evolve into classic ulcers of PG. Superficial granulomatous pyoderma presents as a superficial, localized vegetative or ulcerative lesion that typically follows trauma and responds to less aggressive therapy. Pyostomatitis vegetans is a chronic, vegetative form of PG that can involve the labial and buccal mucosa, most often seen in patients with IBD.

iii. There are no treatments that have demonstrated consistent efficacy in PG. The standard of treatment includes topical, intralesional and/or systemic corticosteroids, depending on the number, size and extent of the lesions. Additional therapies that have been reported in retrospective studies or case series include thalidomide, cyclosporine and clofazimine. The successful use of other therapeutic measures such as immunosuppressants and anti-tumor necrosis factor-alpha (TNF-α) agents have been reported in small case series or case reports.

CASE 34

Granuloma annulare

QUESTION 34

A 45-year-old woman with a history of type II diabetes mellitus presents to the dermatology clinic for enlarging round lesions on the face and arms. She denies any other symptoms and has tried to treat the lesions with topical antifungals due to a concern for a fungal infection. She states this did not help and is concerned about possible transmission to other close contacts. On examination, there are multiple, well-demarcated annular plaques with central clearing on the cheeks and arms with a slightly raised border without evidence of significant scaling (34a, b).

34a

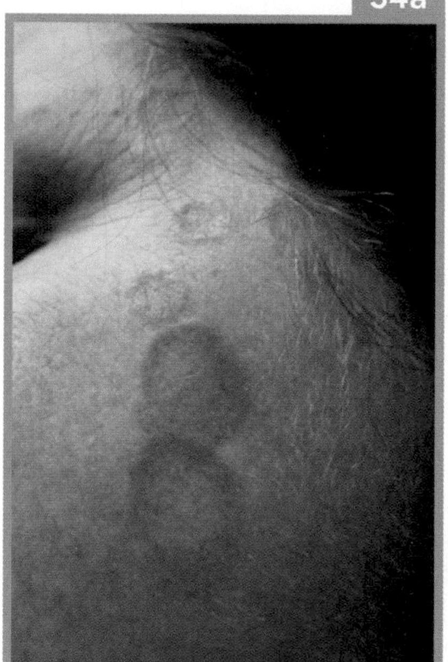

34b

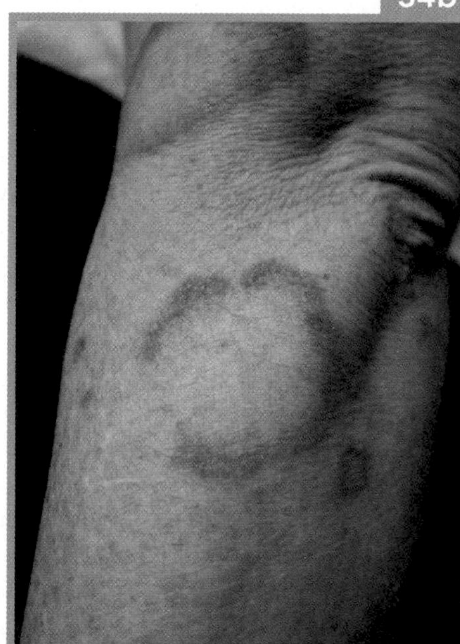

i. What is the diagnosis and is this condition contagious?

ii. What are the characteristic histologic features?

iii. In patients with multiple lesions, what commonly associated metabolic abnormalities can be seen?

Answer 34

i. The patient presents with granuloma annulare (GA), which is a benign, often self-limited disease that presents as small grouped papules forming a plaque in an annular or arcuate configuration. It is seen more commonly in younger patients and in females. Most GA lesions present on the arms and hands, followed by the legs and feet. In a minority of cases, lesions can present simultaneously on the upper and lower extremities, trunk or the face.

Although its appearance can be initially confused with tinea corporis, the raised border of GA can be differentiated from the active border of tinea infections by the presence of small papules at the borders of the GA lesions. In addition, the absence of scaling should suggest GA over tinea. Thus, this patient does not have an infectious process that should prevent her from participating in sports or other activities.

ii. Histologically, GA is a granulomatous dermatitis with focal degeneration of collagen and elastic fibres and mucin deposition. A key finding is the presence of histiocytes, which can be seen in three different patterns. The most common pattern is the interstitial or infiltrative pattern, with histiocytes between collagen fibres, seen in approximately 70% of cases of GA. In the second pattern, palisading granulomas with central connective tissue degeneration and abundant mucin is seen, with surrounding histiocytes and lymphocytes. The third pattern, which is rare, consists of epithelioid histiocytic nodules, which can appear similar to cutaneous sarcoidosis.

iii. In generalized or disseminated GA, nearly half of the cases have been seen in patients with lipid abnormalities, including hypercholesterolemia and/or hypertriglyceridemia. Disseminated GA is also seen in up to one-third of patients with diabetes mellitus. Patients without known diabetes or metabolic abnormalities who present with disseminated GA should undergo evaluation for these conditions. It is important to note that patients with diabetes mellitus are more likely to have chronic relapsing GA than non-diabetics.

CASE 35

Sarcoidosis

QUESTION 35

A 45-year-old African American woman presents to the dermatology clinic with an eruption of bumps on the nose and cheeks. She has been otherwise healthy but was noted to have a serum calcium level of 11.9 mg/dL (reference range: 8.5–10.5 mg/dL) 3 weeks ago on routine laboratory testing at an annual well-adult visit. On examination, there are multiple erythematous, slightly violaceous papules on the nose and cheeks (35).

35

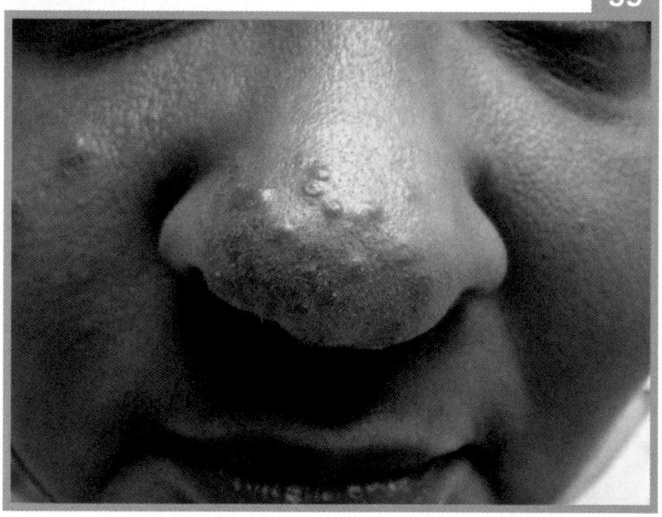

i. What is the most likely diagnosis?

ii. What are important systemic components of this disease?

iii. What is the treatment?

Answer 35

i. The patient's history and presentation is characteristic of lupus pernio, a clinical variant of sarcoidosis. Sarcoidosis, a systemic granulomatous disorder that most commonly affects the lungs, has cutaneous involvement in up to one-third of cases. The skin findings in sarcoidosis consist of red-brown to violaceous papules and plaques that tend to occur on the face, neck, upper trunk, extremities and sites of prior trauma or pre-existing scars. Although sarcoidosis occurs in both men and women of all races and ages, the highest incidence of sarcoidosis has been observed in African American patients in the fourth decade of life.

Laboratory abnormalities that can be seen in sarcoidosis include hypercalcemia (up to 10% of patients), hypercalciuria, lymphopenia, leukopenia and elevated erythrocyte sedimentation rate. Radiologically, asymptomatic hilar and/or paratracheal lymphadenopathy can be found in up to 90% of patients.

ii. As a multisystem disease, sarcoidosis can affect almost any organ, including the lung, heart, liver, spleen, gastrointestinal tract, kidney, bone, eye and central and peripheral nervous systems. Most commonly it affects the lung (up to 90% of patients), ultimately causing fibrosis with bronchiolectasis and honeycombing of the lung parenchyma.

Lupus pernio is important to recognize because patients are more prone to cutaneous scarring and disfigurement, pulmonary and upper respiratory tract involvement, cystic bone lesions and refractory disease.

iii. The mainstay of therapy for systemic sarcoidosis is corticosteroids. Oral prednisone is typically dosed as 1 mg/kg/day for 4–6 weeks, tapered slowly over months to years. Agents that are used to control cutaneous sarcoidosis include intralesional or topical corticosteroids, hydroxychloroquine and chloroquine.

CASE 36

Necrobiosis lipoidica

QUESTION 36

A 64-year-old Caucasian woman with a history of hypertension, rheumatoid arthritis and poorly controlled type II diabetes mellitus presents for evaluation of colour changes on her left foot. She states that it began as a small papule on her foot that grew larger, with some areas of ulceration. Because of her diabetes, she reports decreased sensation throughout her lower extremity. On examination, there is a yellow-brown plaque on the dorsum of her left foot with mild erythema and telangiectasias (36).

36

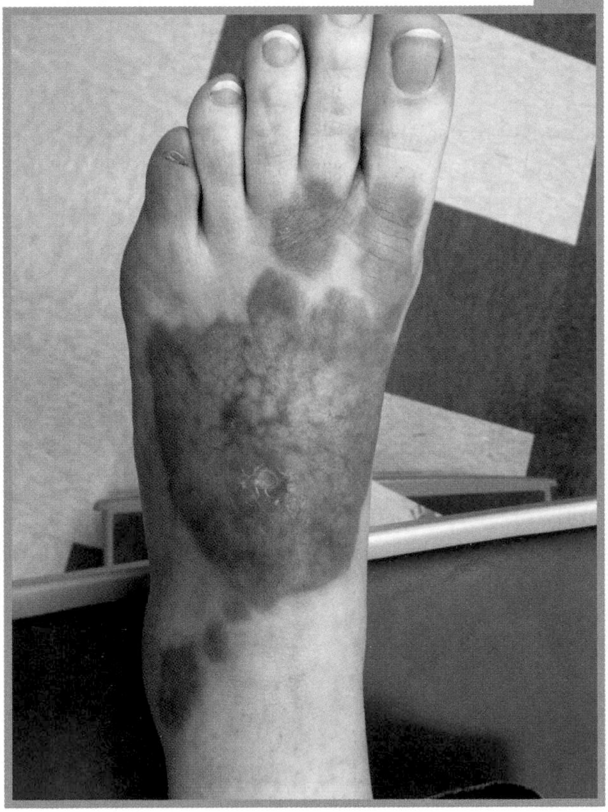

i. What is this disease and what risk factors for this disease does this patient have?

ii. What can be expected on histological examination?

iii. What are treatment options for this disorder?

Answer 36

i. The patient's lesion is necrobiosis lipoidica (NL), previously known as necrobiosis lipoidica diabeticorum. NL is a rare granulomatous disorder that classically presents as a red-brown plaque with a violaceous, raised border and a yellow-brown atrophic centre with scattered telangiectasias. The most common areas of involvement are the distal lower extremities, usually in the pretibial region. Lesions of NL can be multiple and are commonly bilateral and symmetric.

NL has been associated with abnormal glucose metabolism. Although the association is not as prevalent as previously thought, up to 11% of patients with NL have diabetes mellitus at the time of presentation and an additional 11% later develop impaired glucose tolerance or diabetes.

The pathogenesis of NL is poorly understood. The primary cause is thought to be due to immune-mediated vascular disease, as collagen degeneration and dermal inflammation are key findings in NL.

ii. In biopsy specimens taken from the inflammatory border of the lesion, the epidermis may appear normal or atrophic and multiple granulomas throughout the entire dermis can be seen extending to the subcutaneous fat. There may be layered tiers of granulomatous inflammation that lie parallel to the skin surface, around areas of collagen degradation.

iii. Unlike many other cutaneous findings seen in diabetes mellitus, the course of NL does not appear to be affected by the degree of glycemic control and spontaneous resolution is uncommon. NL can be treated with potent topical corticosteroids, with intralesional corticosteroids injected into the active borders of the lesion. Small case series and anecdotal reports suggest the efficacy of niacinamide and antimalarials and for severe, recalcitrant lesions, tumor necrosis factor-alpha (TNF-α) inhibitors have been used with some success.

METABOLIC DISEASES

CASE 37

Gouty tophi

QUESTION 37

A 47-year-old African American man presents to the dermatology clinic with a hard, painful lesion on the right ear. His medical history is notable for hypertension, hyperlipidemia, diabetes mellitus type II, gout and chronic renal insufficiency. He reports that the area on the right ear has been present for several months and when he manipulated it, he was able to express thick white fluid from it. On examination, there is a smooth white papule on the right antihelix with surrounding erythema, which is tender to the touch (37).

37

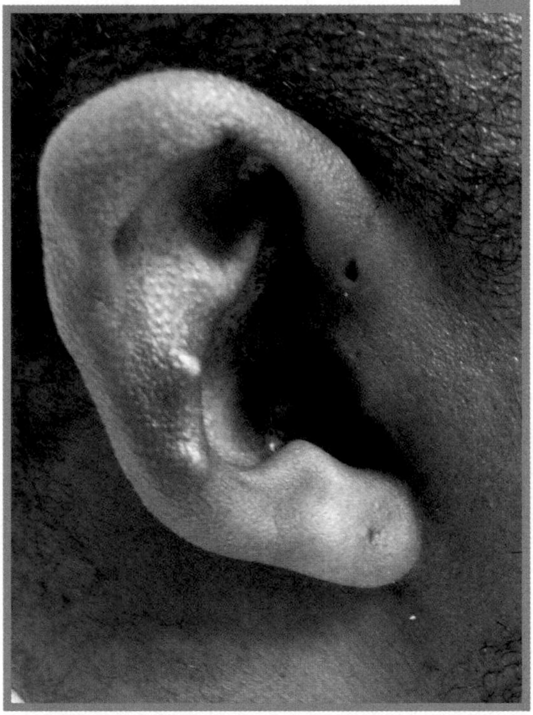

i. What is the underlying cause of this condition?

ii. What are the common risk factors for the development of this cutaneous finding?

iii. What are the characteristic features of this disease on microscopic exam?

iv. What is the treatment of choice?

Answer 37

i. This patient presents with tophaceous gout, which is due to cutaneous deposits of monosodium urate (also known as tophi). Tophi, which are observed in up to 10% of patients with gout, have a predilection for formation on skin overlying joints and the helix of the ear. Clinically, gouty tophi are firm dermal papules or nodules that can vary in color from skin-colored to white–yellow. Occasionally, tophi can become ulcerated and drain white chalky material.

ii. Gouty tophi occur as a result of hyperuricemia. Risk factors for the development of gouty tophi include any processes that result in increased production of uric acid or decreased renal excretion, leading to hyperuricemia. Common risk factors to consider are excessive dietary purine intake, alcohol abuse, conditions of increased nucleotide turnover (such as high-grade lymphomas, myeloproliferative disorders, hemolysis, severe psoriasis), renal insufficiency, diuretic use and drugs such as cyclosporine, tacrolimus, pyrazinamide and low-dose salicylates.

iii. Under polarized light microscope, needle-shaped urate crystals demonstrate negative birefringence. On histopathologic examination, the key features are deposits with needle-like clefts within the dermis and subcutis surrounded by histiocytes and lymphocytes. Crystals in biopsy specimens can be preserved if placed in an ethanol-based fixative such as Carnoy's fluid, in which case refractile brown needle-like crystals can be seen. In silver nitrate solution, the crystals will appear black within yellow surrounding tissue.

iv. The treatment of gouty tophi is directed towards treatment of the underlying gout. In an acute flare, nonsteroidal anti-inflammatory drugs (NSAIDs) such as indomethacin are the therapy of choice. In patients with intolerance or contraindications to NSAIDs, oral colchicine can be used. Urate-lowering therapies such as allopurinol can be used outside of acute gout for prophylaxis.

CASE 38

Acanthosis nigricans

QUESTION 38

A 19-year-old African American woman presents to the dermatology clinic with textural changes and darkly pigmented areas on her neck, elbows and hands. She has no known medical history but her body mass index is 28.5. She reports that she has tried numerous over-the-counter creams and bleaching agents to try to even out the texture and colour, with no improvement. On examination, there are velvety plaques overlying the knuckles and proximal interphalangeal joints of the hands (38), as well as the elbows and the base of the neck.

38

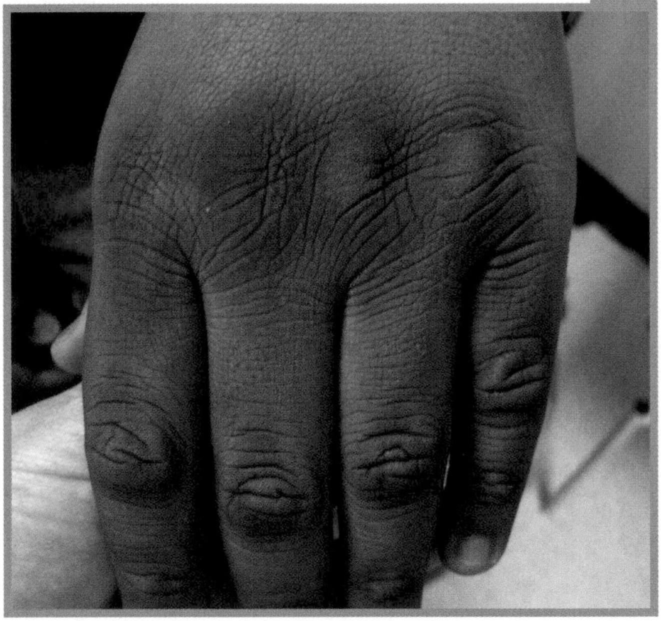

i. What are some of the underlying conditions associated with these findings? What further work-up is appropriate in this patient?

ii. In older individuals, what malignancies can be associated with this cutaneous finding?

Answer 38

i. Acanthosis nigricans (AN) is characterized by velvety hyperpigmentation of the skin that usually involves the flexural areas such as the neck and the axillae, although it can also involve the extensor surfaces such as in this patient. AN is associated most often with insulin resistant states and obesity. It is seen more often in African American and Hispanic patients. AN can also be associated with hyperinsulinemia, Cushing's syndrome, polycystic ovary syndrome (PCOS) and total lipodysrophy. Less often, it can be induced by medications such as systemic corticosteroids, hormone treatments and nicotinic acid. Further history and work-up should be carried out to rule out potential associated diseases such as diabetes mellitus and PCOS.

ii. Malignant AN refers to the disease associated with an internal malignancy. The most commonly associated malignancy is a tumor of the gastrointestinal tract. Malignant AN differs from other forms of AN as it is seen to occur in middle-aged, non-obese patients and can appear abruptly.

CASE 39

Porphyria cutanea tarda

QUESTION 39

A 47-year-old man presents to the emergency department with tense bullae on the hands. He reports that he has had the bullae developing over his hands for approximately 1 month and each lesion starts out as a fluid-filled blister that then denudes and heals with residual scarring. He feels the areas are made worse with sunlight. Upon further questioning he drinks between 6 and 12 cans of beer per night. On physical examination, there are large intact bullae filled with serous fluid on the dorsal aspects of the hands bilaterally on a background of scars from prior lesions (39).

39

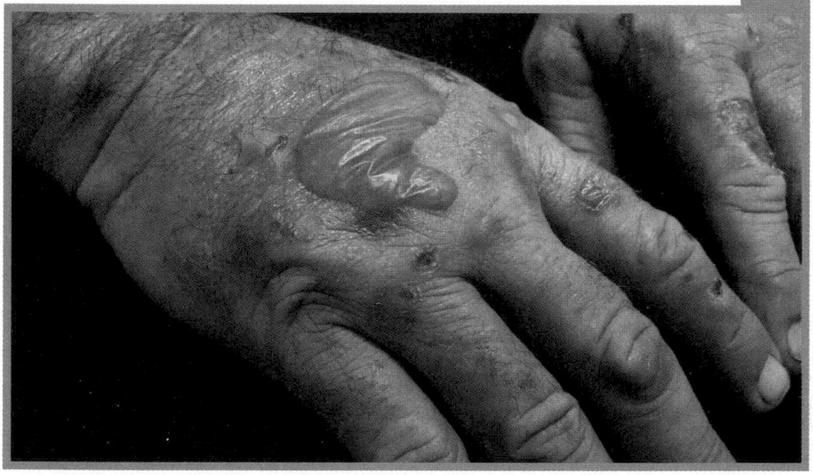

i. What is the diagnosis and how can it be confirmed?

ii. What are some triggers for the development of this condition?

iii. What further laboratory testing and/or screening is indicated in this patient?

iv. What are the treatment options?

Answer 39

i. The patient presents with porphyria cutanea tarda (PCT), which is the most common type of porphyria and is caused by decreased activity of uroporphyrinogen decarboxylase, an enzyme in heme biosynthesis. In the acquired variant, which is seen in this patient, the dysfunctional enzyme is expressed in the liver only. In contrast, in the hereditary variant, the dysfunctional enzyme is observed in all tissues.

PCT is characterized by photosensitivity, skin fragility, blistering, erosions and scars on sun-exposed sites, most often on the dorsal hands and the helices of the ears. The urine of PCT patients will also demonstrate a change in colour to red/brown after several hours of exposure to natural light and will fluoresce pink/red under Wood's lamp/UVA examination. Diagnosis can be confirmed by performing a 24-hour urine collection to measure urine porphyrin levels, which will be elevated. There will also be increased excretion of isocoproporphyrin in the feces.

ii. Known triggers for the development of PCT include alcohol use, oral contraceptives, and viral infections such as hepatitis C and human immunodeficiency virus (HIV).

iii. Further laboratory testing that would be appropriate in a patient with acquired PCT includes a hepatitis panel to evaluate for hepatitis C infection. Additionally, patients with PCT are thought to be at a higher risk of developing hepatocellular carcinoma and screening should be performed in appropriate patient populations.

iv. Treatment options include photoprotection, phlebotomy, hydroxychloroquine and avoidance of triggers.

CASE 40

Scleromyxedema

QUESTION 40

A 56-year-old man presents to the dermatology clinic with an itchy eruption on the ears and neck. They have been present for at least 6 months and seem to be spreading. He also complains of stiffness and thickening of the skin. On physical examination, there are numerous firm, waxy, yellow papules on the posterior ear, postauricular region and posterior neck (40).

40

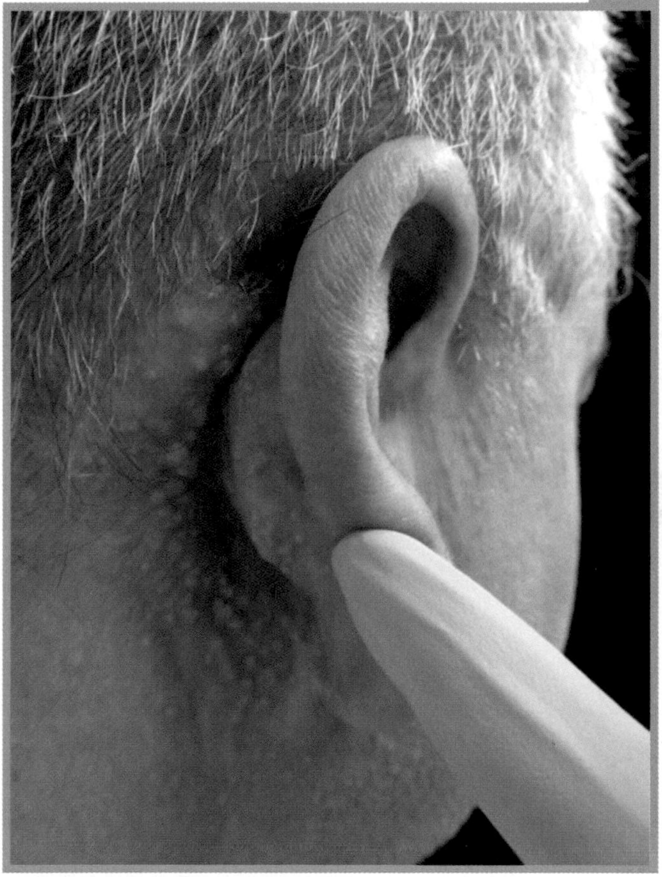

i. What is the most likely diagnosis?

ii. A biopsy was performed to confirm the diagnosis. What are the characteristic findings on histopathological examination?

iii. What additional laboratory work-up or investigation should be considered?

Answer 40

i. This patient presents with scleromyxedema, also known as papular mucinosis. This is an idiopathic cutaneous mucinosis characterized by mucin deposition and increased dermal collagen that can lead to deposition in the skin as well as other internal organs.

Scleromyxedema is seen most often in adults, affecting both men and women equally. It typically present as firm, waxy papules distributed over the head and neck. In some cases, severe involvement can lead to leonine facies due to deposition along the glabella. Internal manifestations of scleromyxedema can lead to neuromuscular, rheumatologic, pulmonary, renal and cardiovascular complications. Systemic symptoms include dysphagia, proximal muscle weakness, peripheral neuropathy, arthropathies, carpal tunnel syndrome, restrictive or obstructive lung disease and renal disease. These may be seen concurrently with cutaneous manifestations or develop later in the disease course.

ii. On histopathological examination, scleromyxedema demonstrates diffuse deposition of mucin in the dermis, increased collagen deposition and proliferation of irregularly arranged fibroblasts. A perivascular infiltrate composed of lymphocytes and plasma cells is often seen.

iii. In almost all cases, scleromyxedema is associated with an immunoglobulin G (IgG) monoclonal gammopathy. Mild plasmacytosis can be seen, but less than 10% of patients will progress to multiple myeloma. However, it is important to further evaluate for the presence of monoclonal gammopathy with additional studies such as basic laboratory tests (complete blood count, comprehensive metabolic panel) and urine and serum protein electrophoresis.

HAIR DISORDERS

CASE 41

Alopecia areata

QUESTION 41

An 11-year-old boy presents to the dermatology clinic with his parents with a 6-month history of progressive hair loss. He feels that larger clumps of hair have been falling out over the past 6 weeks. He remembers having a similar episode several years ago but only had one small patch at that time and never sought treatment. On examination, there are scattered, well-defined patches of alopecia without evidence of scarring (41a, b). On his nails, there is pitting on all 10 fingernails. On trichoscopy, there are yellow dots, black dots and exclamation point hairs within the patches of hair loss.

41a

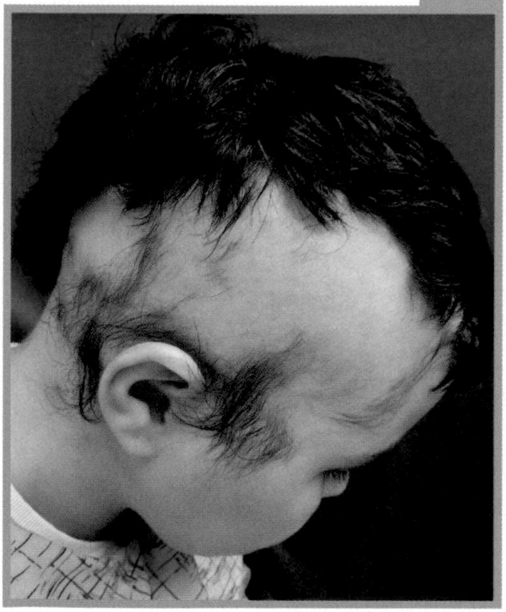

41b

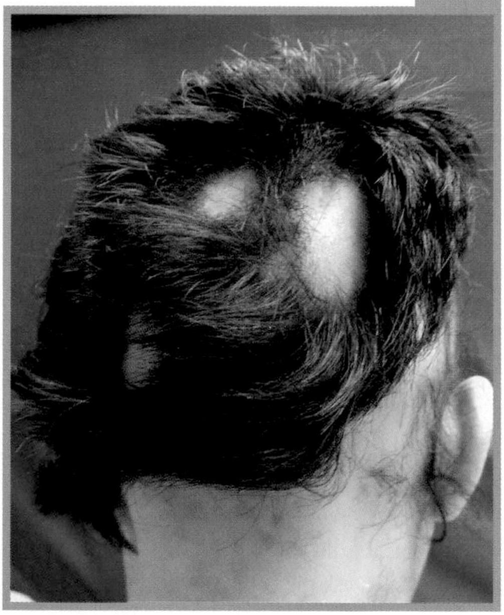

i. What type of alopecia is this?

ii. What further autoimmune work-up should be considered?

iii. What other conditions present with nail pitting?

Answer 41

i. This patient presents with alopecia areata, a non-scarring autoimmune-mediated form of hair loss that typically presents with patchy round or oval areas of hair loss. There are other clinical variants such as alopecia totalis that involves alopecia of all scalp hair, alopecia universalis that involves loss of all scalp and body hair, and alopecia areata with an ophiasis pattern, which consists of band-like hair loss on the occipital and temporal scalp. Examination with trichoscopy will classically reveal yellow to yellow-pink dots, exclamation point hairs and dystrophic hairs.

ii. Alopecia areata is associated with other autoimmune disorders, most commonly with thyroid disease. When evaluating a patient with alopecia areata, it is important to ask screening questions pertinent for thyroiditis such as weight change, change in skin texture, diarrhea, constipation, palpitations and/or fatigue, as well as about family history of autoimmune disease such as lupus erythematosus, myasthenia gravis or rheumatoid arthritis. Further autoimmune work-up with a screening for thyroid stimulating hormone (TSH) level should be considered in patients with clinical signs of thyroid disease.

iii. Conditions that often cause nail pitting include psoriasis, atopic dermatitis, connective tissue disorders and reactive arthritis.

CASE 42

Androgenetic alopecia

QUESTION 42

A 62-year-old woman presents to the dermatology clinic for evaluation of hair loss. She reports that she has noticed progressive thinning of her hair over the last 10 years. She experiences both increased shedding of hair and thinning of hair shafts and does not experience any scalp symptoms such as pruritus, scaling or tenderness. She notes a history of hair loss in her mother and sister. On physical examination, there is generalized thinning on the crown and vertex of the scalp with miniaturization of hair follicles (42).

42

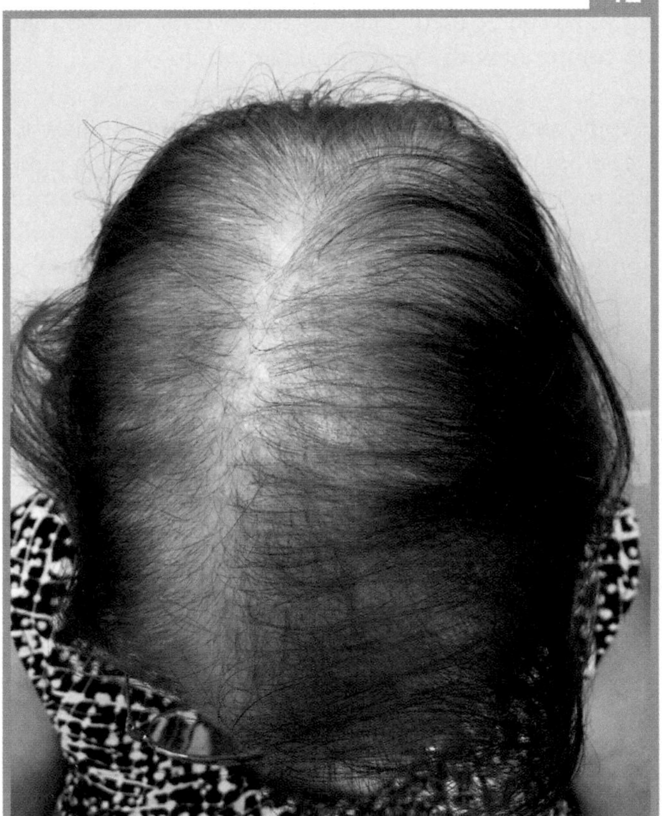

i. What is the diagnosis and what clinical staging systems are available for men and women with this condition?

ii. What are the classic findings on trichoscopy and histologic examination?

iii. What are the treatment options?

Answer 42

i. This patient presents with androgenetic alopecia (AGA), also known as female or male pattern hair loss. AGA is a common, genetically determined condition that leads to miniaturization of hairs over the frontal scalp, crown and vertex. The pathogenesis of AGA is better understood in men and thought to occur as a result of increased type II 5α-reductase and dihydrotestosterone activity in the scalp, which leads to miniaturization of hair follicles and hair shafts. In women, it is thought that there are similar changes in androgen metabolism.

In men, AGA usually affects the frontoparietal scalp and the vertex, in comparison with women, in whom it primarily affects the frontal and parietal scalp. For male pattern hair loss, the Hamilton and Norwood classifications are used to characterize the extent of frontoparietal recession and vertex thinning. In women, the Sinclair and Ludwig scales can be used to classify the severity based on the part width on the frontal scalp compared with the occipital part width.

ii. On trichoscopy, androgenetic alopecia will demonstrate hair shafts of different diameters in more than 20% of hair shafts. Occasionally, a light brown pigment around the hair follicles can also be seen. On histologic examination, these trichoscopic findings are accentuated with a normal total number of hair follicles without significant inflammation but an increased number of vellus hairs.

iii. For mild or early disease, topical treatment with minoxidil 5% can increase hair growth and density. For more advanced disease, systemic medications can be used to slow the progression of AGA. Finasteride, an oral type II 5α-reductase inhibitor, is FDA-approved for the treatment of AGA in men. In women oral finasteride or anti-androgens such as spironolactone and flutamide are used off-label to treat female pattern hair loss. These medications should be used with caution in women of childbearing potential due to the risk of feminization of a male fetus.

CASE 43

Lichen planopilaris

QUESTION 43

A 54-year-old woman presents with progressive hair loss on the crown and vertex of the scalp. She states that this has been ongoing for the past 2–3 years. She notes occasional scalp tenderness, burning and pruritus. On physical examination, there is loss of follicular ostia and increased interfollicular distance on the parietal scalp. There is evidence of perifollicular scaling and inflammation (43a). Two 4-mm punch biopsies were performed, which demonstrated a dense perifollicular lymphocytic infiltrate with wedge-shaped hypergranulosis and perifollicular fibrosis.

43a

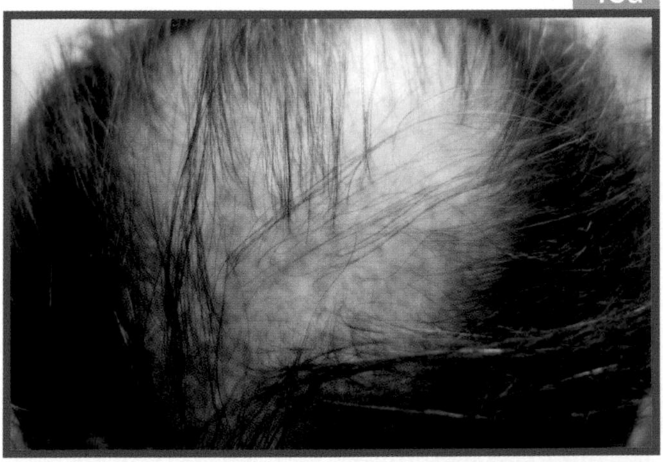

i. What is the diagnosis?

ii. What is another variant of this disease involving the anterior hairline?

iii. What is the treatment of this condition?

Answer 43

i. This patient presents with clinical and histopathologic findings consistent with lichen planopilaris (LPP), a clinical variant of lichen planus with involvement of the hair follicles. Clinically, LPP presents with folliculocentric keratotic plugs with a surrounding erythematous rim on the scalp and other hair-bearing sites. Patients often complain of scalp dysesthesia or a burning sensation, pruritus and tenderness. This variant of lichen planus can lead to permanent scarring and loss of follicular structures and can resemble other causes of end-stage scarring alopecia over time.

ii. Frontal fibrosing alopecia is a more recently recognized variant of LPP, most often seen in older women. It is characterized by progressive hair loss on the frontotemporal hairline and often involves the eyebrows as well (43b). In frontal fibrosing alopecia, there are usually no other signs of lichen planus in the skin or nails.

43b

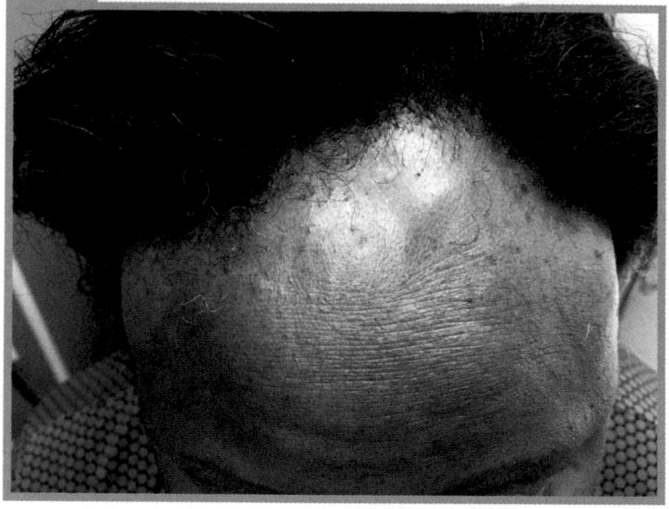

iii. The treatment of lichen planopilaris can include topical and/or intralesional corticosteroids and systemic treatment with agents such as tetracycline antibiotics and hydroxychloroquine.

CASE 44

Folliculitis decalvans

QUESTION 44

A 58-year-old African American man presents to the Veterans Affairs (VA) dermatology clinic for evaluation of recurrent pustules on the scalp and hair loss. This has been ongoing and progressive over the last 10 years. He reports associated scalp symptoms of pruritus, itching, tenderness and burning. He occasionally develops large pus-filled nodules with drainage, with bacterial cultures growing *Staphylococcus aureus* in the past. On examination, there are scattered papules coalescing into plaques on the parietal scalp with areas of patchy, scarring alopecia, with loss of follicular ostia and increased interfollicular distance (44). Two 4-mm punch biopsies are performed, which demonstrates dense perifollicular inflammation in the upper portion of the hair follicles with a mixed inflammatory infiltrate consisting of lymphocytes, neutrophils and plasma cells.

44

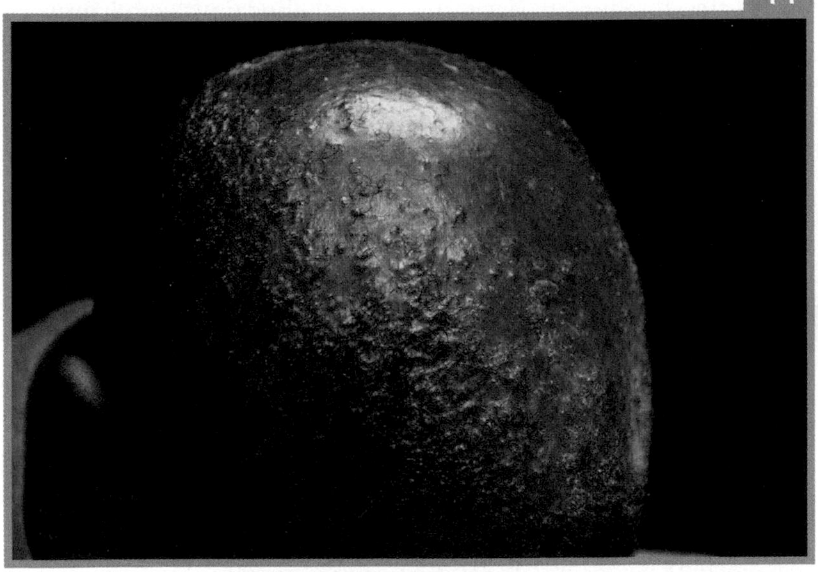

i. What is the most likely diagnosis?

ii. What other forms of hair loss should be included on the differential diagnosis?

iii. Depending on the severity of disease, what treatment options are available?

Answer 14

i. Based on the patient's clinical presentation and histological findings, the most likely diagnosis is folliculitis decalvans, a rare cicatricial or scarring alopecia that affects adolescents and adults. Clinically, folliculitis decalvans presents as inflammatory perifollicular papules and pustules on the scalp with associated scarring alopecia. Superinfection with *S. aureus* is often observed, with some authors hypothesizing a role of a primary *S. aureus* infection of the scalp in the pathogenesis of this disease.

ii. Folliculitis decalvans can appear similar to other scarring forms of hair loss, such as central centrifugal cicatricial scarring alopecia and lichen planopilaris. A skin biopsy can be helpful in distinguishing between these other forms of hair loss. Characteristic features of folliculitis decalvans include a dense perifollicular inflammatory infiltrate confined to the upper third of the follicle, a lymphocytic, neutrophilic or granulomatous inflammatory infiltrate and occasional plasma cells.

iii. For mild cases of folliculitis decalvans, topical clindamycin and antibacterial shampoos can be used to control the inflammation. More severe disease is challenging to treat but first-line therapy involves intralesional corticosteroid injections, oral antibiotics (including tetracyclines, rifampin, ciprofloxacin), and isotretinoin.

DISORDERS OF PIGMENTATION

CASE 45

Vitiligo

QUESTION 45

A 37-year-old man presents to the dermatology clinic for evaluation of spreading pigmentation changes. He reports an 8-month history of progressive lightening of the skin on the hands as well as the face, around the nose and mouth. He denies any history of contact with chemicals or a history of burns. He has no other medical conditions and family history is notable for autoimmune thyroid disease in his mother and type I diabetes in his brother. On examination, there are confluent patches of depigmentation overlying the dorsal hands and wrists with no underlying erythema (45). Examination of the skin under Woods lamp demonstrates enhancement of the depigmented patches with white-blue fluorescence.

45

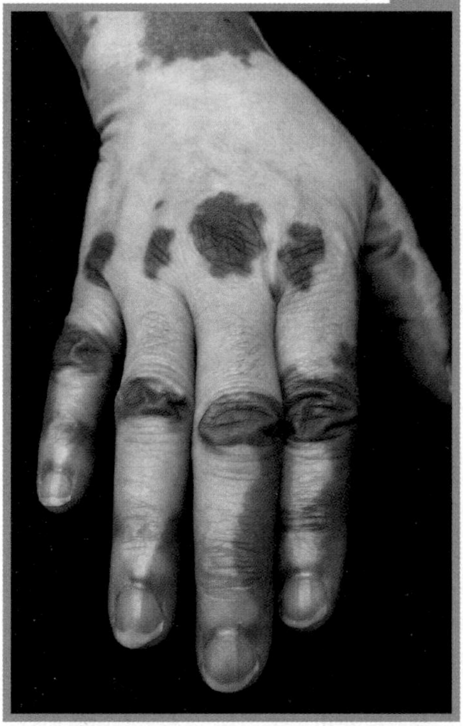

i. What is the diagnosis and what are some associated disorders seen with this disease?

ii. What condition(s) should be considered if the patient had concurrent ocular disease?

iii. What treatment options are available?

Answer 45

i. This patient presents with depigmentation of the skin that is characteristic of vitiligo, an acquired disorder that consists of progressive loss of functional melanocytes, leading to depigmented macules and patches. Although the pathogenesis of vitiligo is not completely understood, it is thought that there may be a genetic component that leads predisposed individuals to develop autoimmune destruction of melanocytes, as well as a possible intrinsic defect in melanocytes that lead to reduced survival and dysregulation of apoptosis.

Vitiligo has a predilection for the head and neck and anatomic regions subject to repeated trauma or friction, such as the hands, wrists, knees and lower legs. On the face, periorificial involvement (around the eyes, nose and mouth) is common. In lightly pigmented individuals, a Wood's lamp can be used to highlight the difference between normally pigmented skin and depigmented areas. Although most cases are asymptomatic, vitiligo can be mildly pruritic and psychosocially challenging to patients.

There are multiple clinical variants of vitiligo. Some lesions of vitiligo are referred to as inflammatory vitiligo due to the presence of a figurate erythematous border at the margin of depigmentation. Trichrome vitiligo describes a patch that consists of an intermediate zone of hypopigmentation between zones of normal pigmentation and depigmentation.

ii. The most significant ocular abnormality associated with vitiligo is uveitis, due to the presence of pigment cells in the uveal tract. Vogt–Koyanagi–Harada syndrome is characterized by uveitis, vitiligo (usually of the head and neck) with poliosis and aseptic meningitis. Alezzandrini syndrome is a rare disease that consists of decreased visual acuity and an atrophic iris associated with depigmentation of the skin on the ipsilateral face as well as poliosis.

iii. The course of vitiligo is unpredictable. It is typically a progressive disease. The goal of treatment is repigmentation and halting disease progression. First-line topical treatments include topical steroids and topical calcineurin inhibitors such as tacrolimus. Repigmentation occurs over the course of months, and occurs in a perifollicular pattern. Other treatments include phototherapy, excimer laser therapy and surgical treatment with autologous transplantation.

CASE 46

Post-inflammatory hyperpigmentation

QUESTION 46

A 66-year-old African American woman presents to the dermatology clinic for follow-up of lichen planus. She has had lichen planus for several years with flares of her disease every 2–3 months. She is currently improved with the use of topical triamcinolone 0.1% ointment. She is concerned about darkly pigmented areas on her arms and back, particularly in areas of the body where lichen planus have resolved. The areas are asymptomatic and have been present for at least 3 months. On examination, there are hyperpigmented macules and patches in a linear arrangement on the left shoulder and upper arm with a well-demarcated border and many scattered hyperpigmented macules on the back, all at sites of prior lichen planus lesions (46a, b).

46a

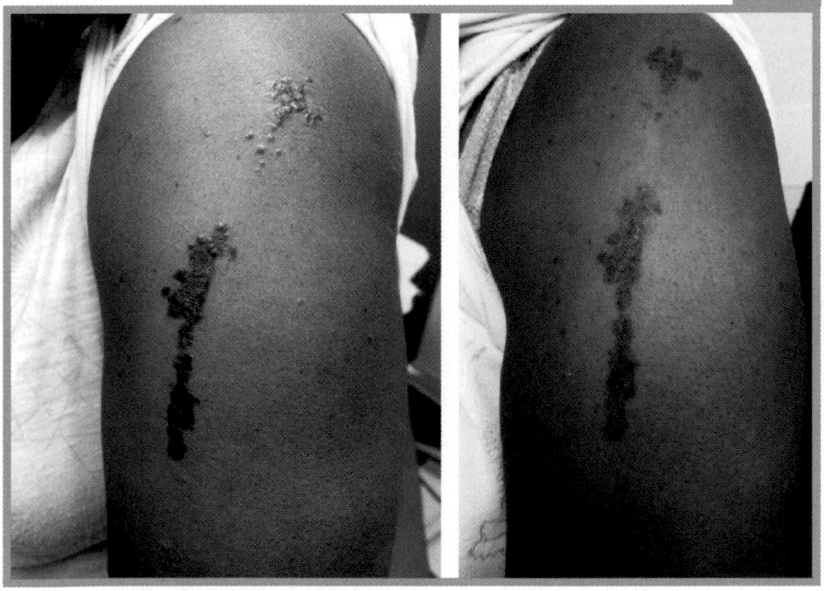

46b

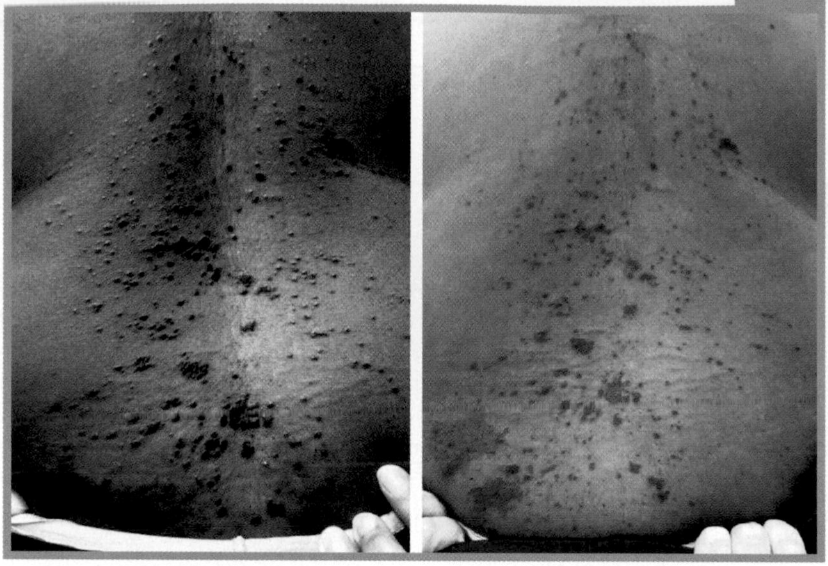

i. What is the diagnosis? In this patient, at what level of the skin does it occur?

ii. What are the treatment options for this patient?

Answer 46

i. This patient presents with post-inflammatory hyperpigmentation (PIH), which is a common dermatologic finding, particularly in individuals with darkly pigmented skin. Post-inflammatory hyperpigmentation is caused by excess melanin pigment deposition after inflammation or injury to the skin. Although in most cases the appearance, distribution and clinical history will direct the clinician to the correct diagnosis, post-inflammatory hyperpigmentation can occur in cases where the preceding inflammation or injury was transient or subclinical.

Epidermal PIH is characterized by tan to brown macules that are usually asymptomatic. Inflammatory mediators such as prostaglandins are thought to enhance pigment production, leading to increased melanin production and transfer to keratinocytes. Common conditions that can lead to epidermal PIH include acne, atopic dermatitis, lichen simplex chronicus, insect bites, psoriasis and lichen planus.

Dermal PIH is characterized by gray-blue to gray-brown pigment changes and is the result of melanin entering the dermis and undergoing phagocytosis by melanophages. It is seen more often in dermatologic conditions that involve inflammation at the dermal–epidermal junction (DEJ), including lichen planus, lichenoid drug reactions and lupus erythematosus.

ii. Epidermal PIH tends to fade over months to years, as long as the primary inflammatory process remains well controlled. Sun protection is an important component of treating epidermal PIH and topical products including hydroquinone, retinoids, corticosteroids, azelaic acid and α-hydroxy acids can be used alone or in combination to help lighten the areas. Dermal PIH can take longer to resolve or may be permanent. Lasers such as Q-switched ruby, alexandrite and neodymium-doped yttrium aluminium garnet (Nd:YAG) have been used with variable success in treating dermal PIH.

CASE 47

Melasma

QUESTION 47

A 36-year-old woman presents to the dermatology clinic for evaluation of dark patches on her face. She states that she has noticed darkening of the skin on the sides of her cheeks after giving birth to her last child approximately 1 year ago. The area is asymptomatic but distressing to her as it is not going away. She recently started taking an oral contraceptive pill but otherwise notes no new medications. Her family history is notable for multiple autoimmune conditions including Grave's disease and systemic lupus erythematosus. She does not wear sunscreen routinely. On examination, there are hyperpigmented patches on the lateral cheeks with areas of hypopigmentation and a reticular pattern on the periphery (47).

47

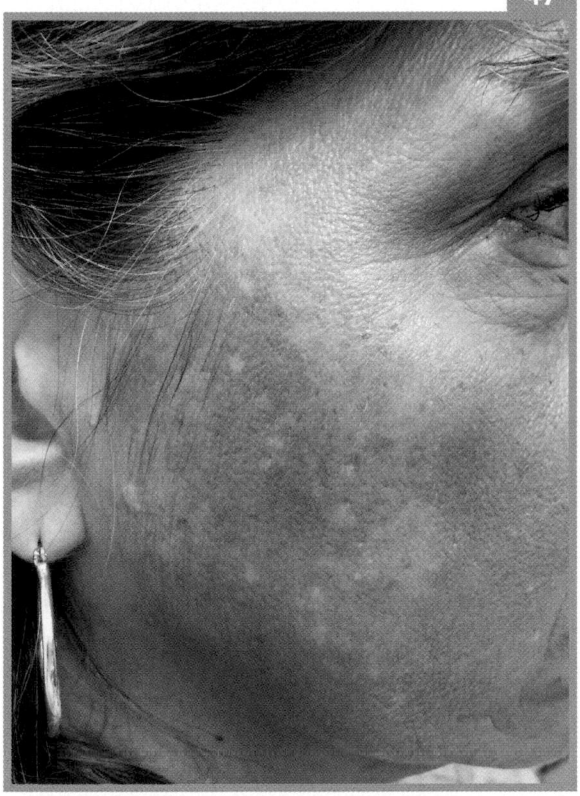

i. What is the diagnosis? What are factors associated with this condition?

ii. What further testing, if any, is indicated?

iii. What treatment options are available?

Answer 47

i. This patient presents with melasma, a common disorder of hyperpigmentation. The classic clinical feature of melasma is the presence of irregular hyperpigmented patches affecting the central face, mandible and/or lateral cheeks. Although the exact pathogenesis of melasma is not fully understood, there are several well known risk factors associated with this condition, including genetic predisposition, darker skin types (Fitzpatrick skin type III and higher), exposure to UV light, pregnancy and exogenous hormones such as oral contraceptives or hormone replacement therapy.

ii. Thyroid disorders can be associated with melasma. Given this patient's age and family history, it would be prudent to perform baseline screening for any thyroid dysfunction.

iii. Melasma can be challenging to treat. Although there is no single treatment that has demonstrated uniform efficacy in large-scale studies, combination therapy with multiple treatments appears to be the most effective approach. Topical treatments should include the use of a broad-spectrum sunscreen to prevent worsening of melasma. Other topical medications include hydroquinone, mequinol, tretinoin, adapalene and mild topical corticosteroids. Chemical peels with alpha hydroxy peeling agents such as glycolic acid can also improve hyperpigmentation by removing unwanted melanin, but should be used with caution as over-irritation can lead to post-inflammatory hyperpigmentation. Laser therapy can also be beneficial in select patients with melasma, depending on their Fitzpatrick skin types. Various lasers such as Q-switched ruby lasers have been shown to worsen melasma, while intense pulsed light therapy may provide some benefit as an adjunctive therapy.

NEOPLASMS OF THE SKIN

CASE 48

Pyogenic granuloma

QUESTION 48

A 14-year-old girl presents to the dermatology clinic for evaluation of a rapidly growing lesion on her chin. The patient recalls a possible mosquito bite to the area a week before developing a small red bump. The area has grown over the last 4 weeks and is easily traumatized and bleeds. On examination, there is an exophytic, bright red papule on the left chin (48).

48

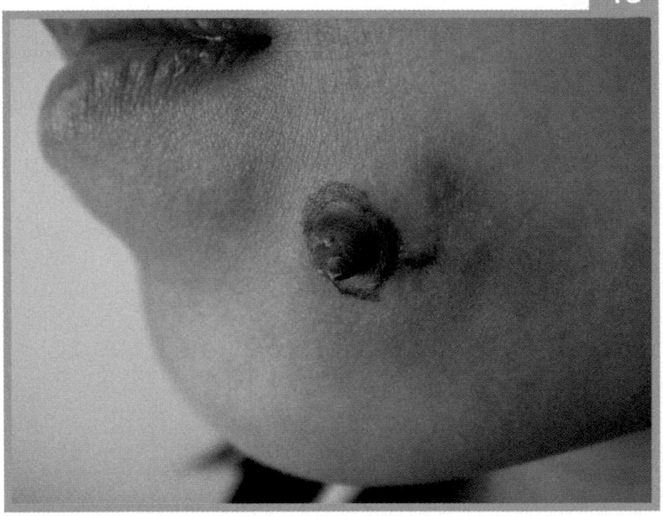

i. What is the most likely diagnosis and what other conditions should be included on the differential diagnosis?

ii. What medications can be associated with this condition?

iii. What is the treatment of choice?

Answer 48

i. This patient presents with a pyogenic granuloma, also known as a lobular capillary hemangioma. These are benign neoplasms that are thought to occur through a process of reactive neovascularization. Pyogenic granulomas are most often observed in children and young adults and commonly occur after minor trauma. The lesions have a predilection for the gingiva, fingers, lips, face and tongue. They often develop as a solitary papule that can grow rapidly over weeks to months. Patients often report that the lesions bleed easily with minor trauma.

Additional considerations in the differential diagnosis of a bright red bleeding papule include amelanotic melanoma, bacillary angiomatosis, Kaposi's sarcoma, glomus tumors, hemangiomas and irritated nevi or warts.

ii. Pyogenic granulomas occur in association with medications, including systemic retinoids, indinavir and epidermal growth factor receptor (EGFR) inhibitors.

iii. The treatment of choice for pyogenic granulomas is shave excision with electrosurgery of the base. Recurrence after removal is possible. In small pyogenic granulomas, successful treatment with pulsed dye laser and sclerotherapy has been reported in few cases.

CASE 49

Actinic keratosis

QUESTION 49

An 87-year-old woman presents to the dermatology clinic for a routine total body skin examination. She has a history of chronic sun exposure and spends much of her time gardening. She has noted development of crusty papules on her hands and arms. The papules have grown in size over the last 6 months and occasionally flake off and bleed. On examination, there are erythematous hyperkeratotic papules symmetrically distributed over the dorsal hands and forearms (49).

49

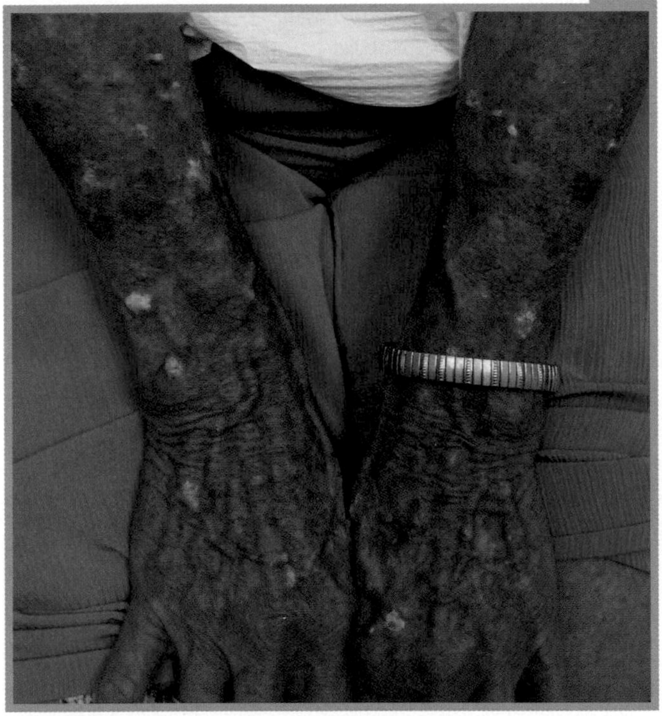

i. What skin lesions does this patient have?

ii. What different therapies are available for these lesions?

iii. What subset of immunosuppressed patients are at higher risk for these neoplasms?

Answer 49

i. This patient is presenting with multiple hypertrophic actinic keratoses (AKs). Actinic keratoses are common epithelial precancerous lesions that can be classified into different categories based on their pathogenesis. The most common are ultraviolet (UV)-induced, human papillomavirus (HPV)-induced and arsenic-induced. Because of the distribution of lesions, patient's age and the patient's history of cumulative sun exposure, she is most likely presenting with numerous solar or UV-induced actinic keratoses. AKs are usually hyperkeratotic and rough on palpation, may have varying degrees of erythema and can be pigmented.

Although AKs are considered to be precancerous, they serve as a risk marker for skin cancer and have the capacity to progress into squamous cell carcinomas (SCC). The transformation rate from AK to SCC is considerably low, ranging from 0.1% to 0.24%, but the rate of concurrent AK and invasive SCC is between 5% and 20%. Furthermore, 84%–100% of patients with invasive SCC on UV-exposure of the skin also have a history of AKs.

ii. There are various treatments available for actinic keratoses. Physical treatment options include cryotherapy with liquid nitrogen, curettage and electrocoagulation, laser therapies and photodynamic therapy. Topical treatment options are also available, which include 5-fluorouracil with or without salicylic acid, imiquimod, diclofenac sodium and ingenol mebutate.

iii. Organ transplant recipients are a subset of patients with a higher risk of developing AKs and eventually SCCs, with almost a 100-fold higher incidence than in the general population. It is also thought that AK lesions in this population tend to follow a more aggressive clinical course, with a more rapid progression to SCC. Close monitoring and aggressive treatment is necessary in these patients.

CASE 50

Basal cell carcinoma

QUESTION 50

A 68-year-old woman presents to the dermatology clinic for evaluation of a new growth on the right nasal wall. She states that it has been present for approximately 6 months, has grown, is tender to the touch and occasionally bleeds with minimal trauma. On examination, there is a pearly papule with a slightly rolled border and branching telangectasias throughout the lesion (50).

50

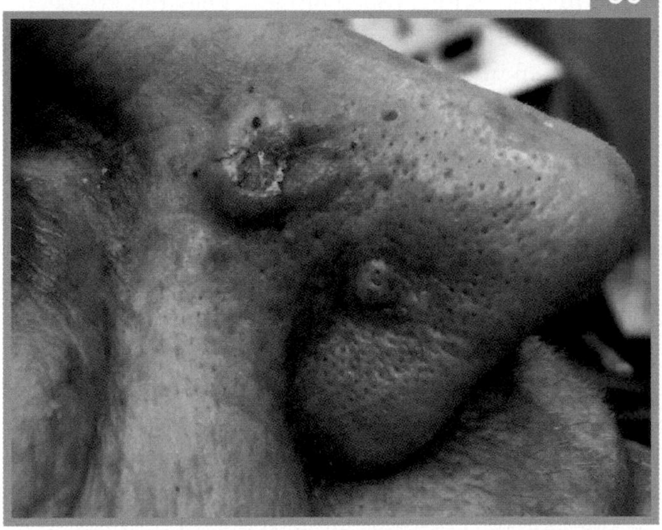

i. What is the diagnosis?

ii. What are the four major clinicopathological variants of this neoplasm?

iii. What different therapies are available for these lesions?

Answer 50

i. This patient presents with basal cell carcinoma (BCC), the most common non-melanoma skin cancer (NMSC) observed in Caucasian individuals. Up to 75%–80% of NMSCs are BCCs and up to 20%–25% are SCCs. The major risk factors for developing a BCC are UV exposure either from intermittent sun exposure or other exposures to UV light, such as from tanning beds.

ii. Although there are numerous subtypes of BCCs, the four major clinicopathologic types are (1) nodular, (2) superficial, (3) morpheaform and (4) fibroepithelial BCC. The most common form is the nodular type, which accounts for about 50% of BCCs and is characterized clinically by a pearly papule or nodule with arborizing telangiectasias. Nodular BCCs also demonstrate a higher tendency to grow larger and ulcerate with a rolled border. They tend to occur on the face, particularly on the cheeks, nose, forehead and eyelids, but can also be seen on any hair-bearing sites. Superficial BCCs tend to grow horizontally and are less likely to develop into nodules with induration and ulceration. They are characterized by erythematous macules or thin papules, with occasionally a thin rolled border. Morpheaform BCCs are an uncommon subtype and often appear as a light pink to white area of induration that is ill-defined and can resemble a scar or morphea. This variant tends to behave more aggressively and can lead to local destruction. Fibroepithelial BCC is a rare variant that tends to occur on the trunk. It presents as a skin-coloured or pink papule with a smooth surface.

iii. Depending on the clinicopathologic type, location and size of the cancer, there are various treatment options available. For small, superficial cancers, cryosurgery, photodynamic therapy and medical treatment with topical application of 5-fluorouracil or imiquimod can be used. Surgical procedures include curettage with electrodesiccation, standard surgical excision and Mohs micrographic surgery. Highest cure rates are observed with Mohs micrographic surgery.

CASE 51

Squamous cell carcinoma

QUESTION 51

A 72-year-old woman with a history of mild Alzheimer's disease presents with a new growth on her arm. The lesion has developed over several months, is painful and itchy. She has had multiple seborrheic keratoses treated with cryotherapy in the past and has a history of significant sun exposure with a background of chronic photodamage. On examination, there is an erythematous papule with a central keratotic core located on the forearm (51).

51

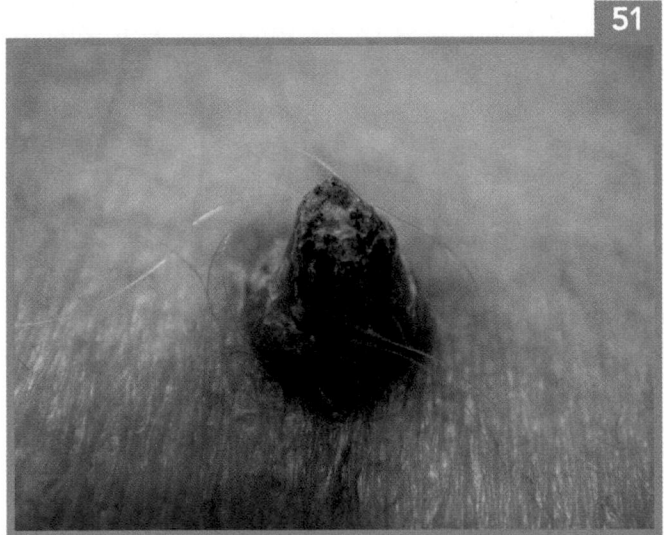

i. What is the most likely diagnosis?

ii. What are the classic histologic findings in this lesion?

iii. What are the risk factors for metastasis?

iv. What is the most appropriate treatment modality?

Answer 51

i. The patient presents with a lesion indicative of cutaneous squamous cell carcinoma (SCC). SCCs often arise in elderly individuals on areas of chronic sun exposure. They can present with wide variation, but the appearance of this patient's lesion is consistent with an exophytic, hyperkeratotic SCC.

Staging of SCC is performed based on the tumour, lymph node and metastases (TNM) cancer staging system, taking into account the size of the tumour and depth of invasion. Although most SCCs that arise on areas of chronic sun exposure tend to be early-stage diseases, lesions involving special sites such as the lips, vulva and penis are associated with a higher risk of aggressive tumour behaviour.

ii. In well-differentiated invasive SCCs, keratin pearls with atypical keratinocytes at varying level of the dermis are seen. In poorly differentiated SCCs, strands and cords of epithelial cells with prominent nuclear atypia can be seen without signs of keratinization. There can also be perineural growth, neurotropism and atypical keratinocytes with acantholysis.

iii. Metastases are seen in approximately 5% of invasive SCCs. Risk factors for metastasis of invasive SCCs include: tumour thickness >2 mm; diameter >2 cm; location on the ears, lips, tongue, vulva or penis; arising within a scar from a burn or radiation injury; poorly differentiated or undifferentiated SCC on histopathology and immunosuppressed individual.

iv. Surgical excision is the treatment of choice for invasive SCCs. High-risk SCCs require excision with 6-mm margins. Recurrence at the same site is possible, and these patients are at higher risk of developing further non-melanoma skin cancers (NMSCs). Thus, patients should thereafter undergo routine dermatologic screening.

CASE 52

Keratoacanthoma

QUESTION 52

A 62-year-old woman with a history of depression and hypothyroidism presents with a new lesion that has rapidly evolved over several weeks. It started as a small red papule on the forearm but developed into a nodule with a central crater. She denies any associated pain or tenderness, but states it bothers her due to its location and size. On examination, there is a well-circumscribed nodule with a central hyperkeratotic core (52).

52

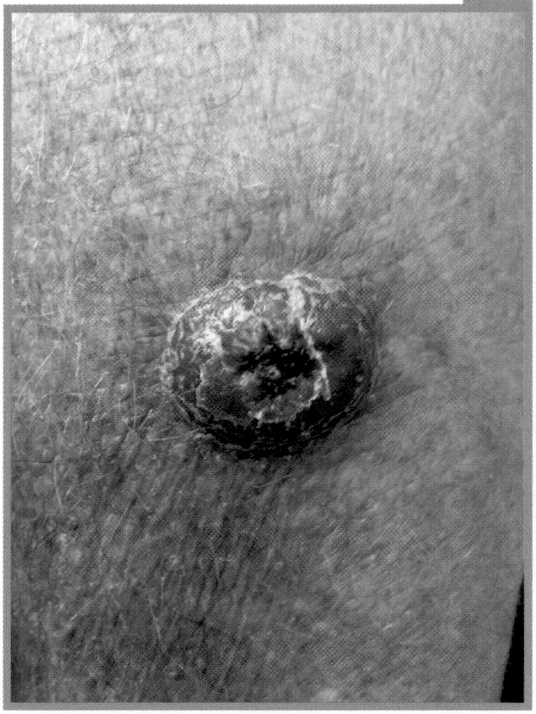

i. Given the appearance and time course, what is the most likely diagnosis?

ii. What is the characteristic histologic finding in this lesion?

iii. What are potential treatment options for this lesion?

iv. What is the variant characterized by the generalized eruption of these lesions in an adult?

Answer 52

i. The appearance and time course of the lesion is consistent with keratoacanthoma (KA). Although there are some who consider KAs to be a variant of squamous cell carcinomas, others consider KAs to be benign tumours. KAs commonly present as solitary lesions that range in size from 5–15 mm in diameter with a predilection for the head and neck region or sun-exposed skin. KAs can also present as multiple, grouped or giant lesions. One clinical variant, known as keratoacanthoma centrifugum marginatum, can be as large as several centimeters in diameter and heal with prominent atrophic scarring. Ferguson–Smith syndrome is an autosomal dominant condition in which multiple spontaneously regressing KAs develop in the third decade of life.

ii. Histologically, KAs typically have a dome-shaped architecture, made up of well-differentiated keratinocytes with a brightly eosinophilic glassy cytoplasm and minimal cytologic atypia. The core of the KA is filled with cornified material and an inflammatory infiltrate.

iii. KAs usually regress spontaneously, but a skin biopsy is often performed to establish the diagnosis and rule out squamous cell carcinoma. KAs can be treated with excision, electrodessication and curettage, with or without cryosurgery with liquid nitrogen or photodynamic therapy. Intralesional treatment with 5-fluorouracil or methotrexate has also been reported as effective in the treatment of KAs.

iv. Generalized eruptive keratoacanthoma, also known as the Gryzbowski type, is characterized by the sudden eruption of hundreds to thousands of small (typically 2–3 mm) keratoacanthoma over the entire body, including the palms, soles, larynx and oral mucosa. Given the disseminated nature of this variant, it is often treated with systemic therapies such as oral retinoids, methotrexate, 5-fluorouracil and cyclophosphamide.

CASE 53

Melanoma

QUESTION 53

A 51-year-old man presents to the dermatology clinic for an annual skin examination. He has no personal history of skin cancer but reports a history of multiple 'abnormal moles' that required removal throughout his adolescence and into early adulthood. He has a history of significant sun exposure over his lifetime and does not wear sunscreen. His family history is notable for skin cancer in his paternal grandmother. On examination, there is a red-brown slightly raised melanocytic papule with asymmetry and irregular pigmentation at the border (53a). Under dermatoscopy, the lesion demonstrates asymmetry, a scar-like depigmentation in the centre with an irregular pigment network and multiple colours (white, tan, red, brown) (53b).

53a

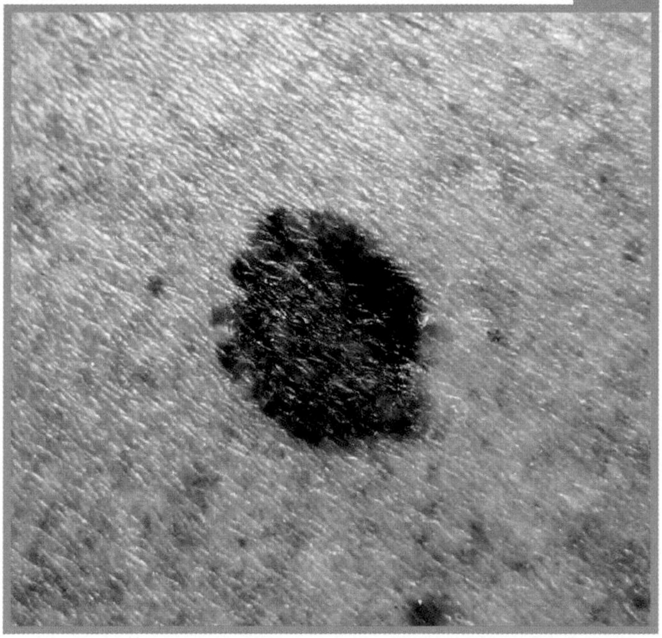

53b

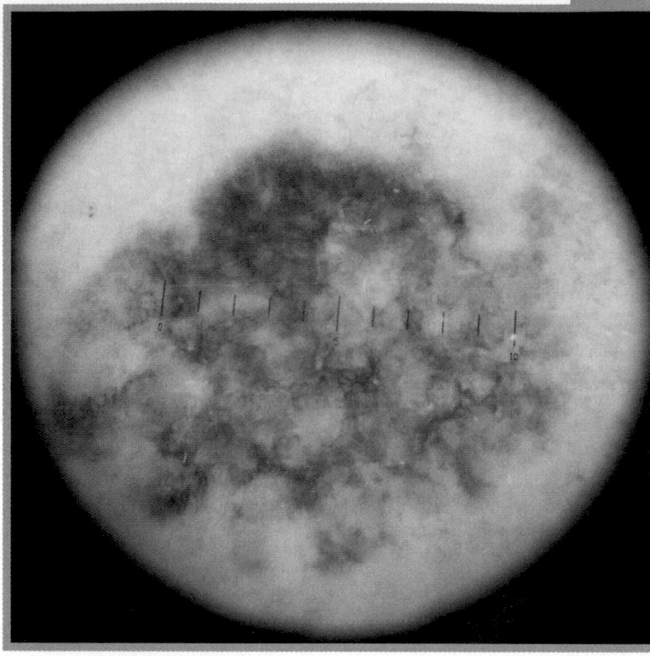

i. What is the diagnosis, and what are the risk factors for developing this skin lesion?

ii. What are the four major variants of this condition?

iii. What are the histologic characteristics of this lesion, and what stains can help confirm the diagnosis?

iv. What are the molecular targeted therapies available for advanced disease?

Answer 53

i. The patient presents with a melanocytic lesion with clinical and dermatoscopic features that are consistent with malignant melanoma, a malignant tumour of melanocytes. The incidence of melanoma has increased in Caucasian populations worldwide and is responsible for >75% of skin cancer deaths.

There are many risk factors for the development of melanoma. Genetic factors include a family history of melanoma, lightly pigmented skin with a tendency towards sunburn, red hair colour and any underlying DNA repair defects such as xeroderma pigmentosum. Environmental factors also contribute to the development of cutaneous melanoma and include a history of chronic sun exposure or intense intermittent sun exposure, a history of psoralen and ultraviolet A radiation (PUVA) therapy, use of tanning beds, and immunosuppression. In patients with large congenital melanocytic nevi (>20 cm in diameter), there is a higher risk for developing melanoma than in normal melanocytic nevi.

ii. The four types of primary melanomas, categorized by their growth patterns, include: (1) superficial spreading melanoma (most common, comprise >50% of primary cutaneous melanoma), (2) nodular melanoma, (3) lentigo maligna and (4) acral lentiginous melanoma. There are also numerous other variants of melanoma, defined by clinical or histologic features, such as amelanotic melanoma, spitzoid melanoma, and desmoplastic melanoma, among others.

iii. On histology, melanomas can demonstrate a wide variety of features. Some of the key criteria for the histopathologic diagnosis of melanoma include asymmetry, poor circumscription, a lack of maturation of melanocytes, confluent nests of melanocytes that vary in size and shape, dyshesive melanocytic nests, atypical melanocytes with the presence of mitotic figures and signs of regression of the lesion. In addition, immunohistochemical stains can aid in the diagnosis of melanoma. Human melanoma black 45 (HMB-45) is a stain that can identify tumour cells of melanocytic lineage, and S100 is a stain that is highly sensitive for melanocytes and melanoma, although it is not specific.

iv. For patients with metastatic disease, the 5-year survival rate remains around 10% and the mainstay of therapy is systemic treatment with chemotherapy, immunotherapy or combined biochemotherapy. Tumour genotyping studies have demonstrated that up to 60% of melanomas have an activating mutation in B-Raf murine sarcoma viral oncogene homolog B1 (*BRAF*) and a smaller proportion have mutations in the *KIT* receptor gene. Vemurafenib is a selective BRAF inhibitor that has demonstrated mortality benefits when used in patients with metastatic melanoma carrying a specific point mutation in *BRAF*. There are some reports supporting the use of KIT inhibitors such as imatinib and dasatinib for the treatment of patients with melanoma with mutations in the *KIT* receptor gene, but these drugs are still undergoing clinical trials.

CASE 54

Trichoepithelioma

QUESTION 54

A 54-year-old woman presents to the dermatology clinic as a referral from her otolaryngologist for the evaluation of a growing tumour on and around the left ear. She is unsure of how long the tumour has been present. On examination, there is a pink nodular plaque involving the tragus and spanning from the antitragus to the crus of the helix (54). On histology, there are basaloid islands in a sclerotic stroma with concentric collagen and many fibroblasts.

54

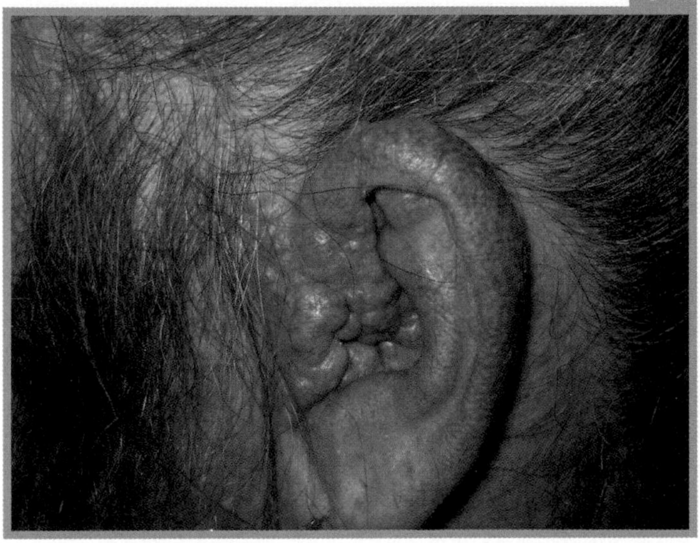

i. What is the diagnosis?

ii. What is the inheritance pattern of this condition? What syndrome(s) is/are associated with this growth?

iii. What is the other variant of this tumour, and what is the pitfall in its diagnosis and management?

Answer 54

i. The patient presents with clinical and histological findings of a trichoepithelioma, a benign neoplasm of follicular germinative differentiation. Classic trichoepitheliomas present as skin-coloured papules or nodules on the face or upper trunk.

ii. Multiple trichoepitheliomas, known as epithelioma adenoids cysticum, can be seen associated with familial cylindromatosis, an autosomal dominant condition caused by a mutation in the cylindromatosis (*CYLD*) gene. In addition, there are several syndromes associated with multiple trichoepitheliomas, listed below.

Syndrome	Cutaneous findings
Brooke–Spiegler syndrome	Multiple cylindromas and trichoepitheliomas
Rombo syndrome	Multiple trichoepitheliomas, milia, vermiculate atrophy, basal cell carcinoma, peripheral vasodilation and cyanosis
Rasmussen's syndrome	Multiple trichoepitheliomas, cylindromas and milia

iii. The desmoplastic variant of trichoepitheliomas can demonstrate histologic features indistinguishable from those of basal cell carcinomas, such as peripheral palisading and a sclerotic stroma.

CASE 55

Telangiectasia macularis eruptiva perstans

QUESTION 55

A 56-year-old man presents to the dermatology clinic for a routine skin check. On examination, there are small erythematous telangiectatic macules ranging in size from 3 to 10 mm distributed on the face, shoulders, upper arms and back (55a). With friction, the areas become slightly papular. There is no palpable lymphadenopathy or hepatosplenomegaly. He denies any fever, chills, abdominal pain or other skin concerns. Upon further questioning, the patient states that the symptoms have been evolving over the past 2 years. A skin biopsy was performed, which revealed a mononuclear infiltrate consisting of mast cells surrounding the capillaries of the superficial dermis. All laboratory work-up including a peripheral blood smear are within normal limits.

55a

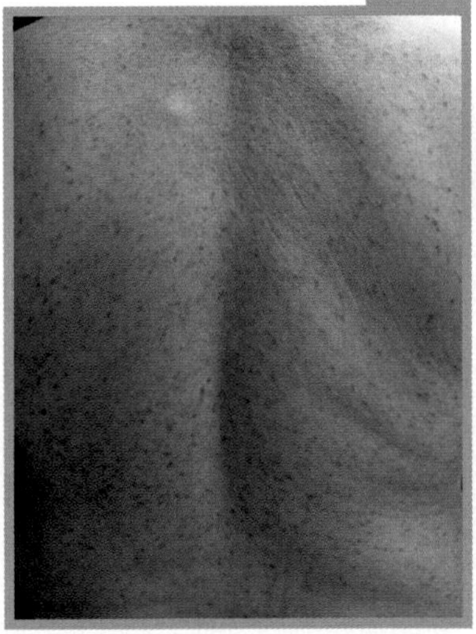

i. What is the most accurate diagnosis for this patient?

ii. What are the names of the cutaneous forms of mastocytosis, and what are the most common forms in children?

iii. What is the name of the clinical sign elicited at the site of friction in patients with cutaneous mastocytosis?

iv. What stain can help confirm the presence of mast cells?

v. What mutation is commonly seen in mastocytosis?

Answer 55

i. The most accurate diagnosis is telangiectasia macularis eruptiva perstans (TMEP), which is an uncommon form of adult cutaneous mastocytosis. It is characterized by telangiectatic macules and patches without significant hyperpigmentation. Additional clinical findings include a doughy consistency of the skin and in more advanced stages, skinfolds can become thickened and lead to disfigurement.

ii. The cutaneous forms of mastocytosis include solitary mastocytoma, urticaria pigmentosa (UP) and diffuse cutaneous mastocytosis. Mastocytomas and UP are the most common forms in children. Mastocytomas are usually solitary plaques or nodules with yellow-tan or brown colour that can be present at birth or develop during infancy. UP consists of macules and papules with varying degrees of hyperpigmentation that favour the trunk and spare the face, palms and soles (55b). Diffuse cutaneous mastocytosis, which is a rare form in children, presents with erythematous yellow-tan papules and plaques with a leathery texture.

55b

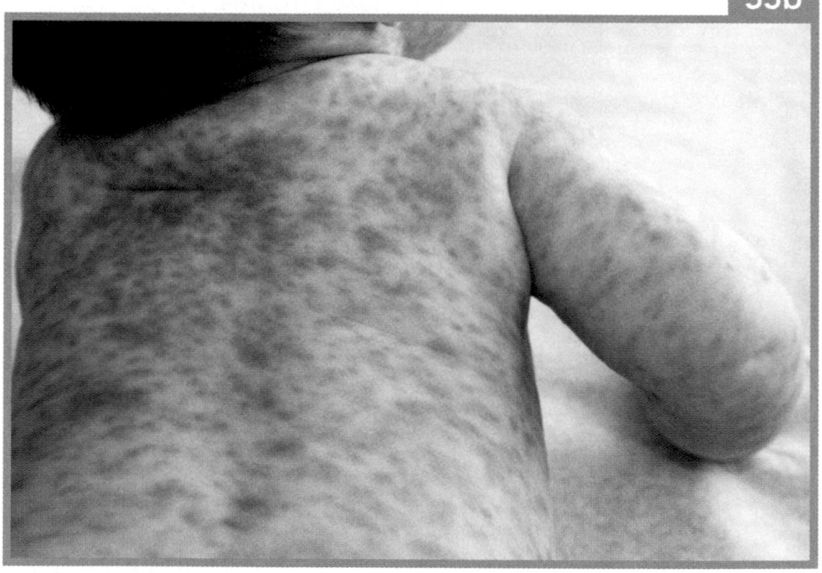

iii. In patients with mast cell hyperplasia in the skin due to mastocytosis, rubbing the skin will elicit the formation of an urticarial wheal, also known as Darier's sign. The development of an urticarial wheal confirms mast cell mediator release and is seen more prominently in mastocytomas and UP in childhood, while often less apparent in adult mastocytosis lesions or TMEP. The extent of this clinical sign is thought to reflect mast cell concentrations in the skin. In mastocytomas and childhood UP, mast cell concentrations are reportedly

40 to 150-fold higher than in normal skin, compared to only 8-fold higher in the skin of adult mastocytosis patients.

iv. Immunohistochemical staining for KIT (CD117) can help confirm the diagnosis of mastocytosis.

v. The most common mutation seen in mastocytosis is a somatic mutation of codon 816 of the *c-KIT* proto-oncogene located on chromosome 4q12. This mutation leads to constitutive activation of the KIT tyrosine kinase receptor.

CASE 56

Cutaneous B-cell lymphoma

QUESTION 56

A 47-year-old woman presents to the dermatology clinic as a referral from her primary care physician for evaluation of skin lesions on her forehead. They have been present for 8–9 months. Prior treatments with topical corticosteroids and topical antimicrobial washes have proven ineffective in eradicating the lesions. The lesions have been relatively asymptomatic throughout their course, but she does not like the appearance of the lesions. She does not note any other areas of involvement. On examination, there are multiple red-brown papules and nodules on the left forehead with no overlying skin changes (56). No lymphadenopathy was noted and the remainder of the physical examination was unremarkable. On review of systems, the patient denied weight loss, fatigue, malaise, fever or chills. A biopsy was performed to confirm the diagnosis.

56

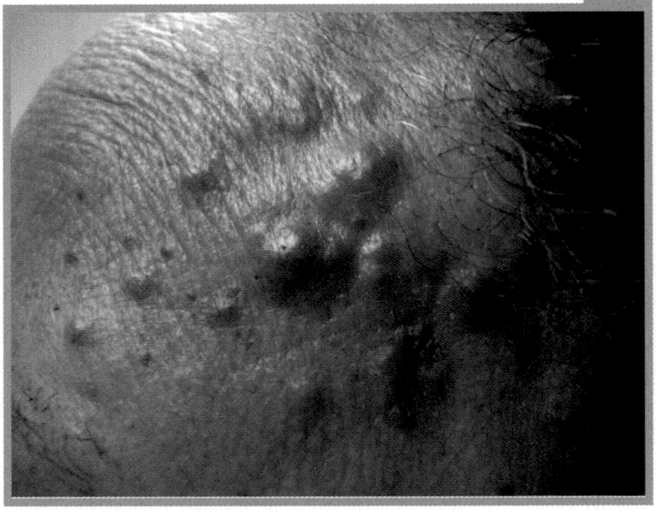

i. What is the most likely diagnosis?

ii. What are the other clinical and laboratory findings that support this diagnosis and what additional testing, if any, should be performed?

iii. What are the characteristic features of this disease on histopathological examination?

iv. What is the prognosis? What are the treatment options?

Answer 56

i. This patient most likely has a primary cutaneous B-cell lymphoma (pCBCL), which represents 22.5% of all cutaneous lymphomas according to the World Health Organization (WHO) and the European Organization for Research and Treatment of Cancer (EORTC). There are four major types of pCBCL, which include (1) primary cutaneous follicle centre lymphoma, (2) primary cutaneous marginal zone B-cell lymphoma, (3) primary cutaneous diffuse large B-cell lymphoma (leg type) and (4) intravascular diffuse large B-cell lymphoma.

The patient's cutaneous findings are most consistent with primary cutaneous follicle centre lymphoma, which is a common subtype of pCBCL. It is characterized by red-violaceous papules and plaques or tumours commonly located on the scalp, forehead or back. Ulceration, pain or other symptoms are rarely observed. These tumours grow in an indolent course and less than 10% of the patients have involvement of extracutaneous sites.

Primary cutaneous marginal zone B-cell lymphoma is characterized by the recurrent red-brown papules, plaques and nodules that tend to occur on the extremities or trunk. Similar to primary cutaneous follicle centre lymphoma, ulceration or associated symptoms are rarely observed. This subtype of pCBCL has been linked to infection by *Borrelia*. Primary cutaneous diffuse large B-cell lymphoma (leg type) presents with erythematous nodules on the distal legs that may become ulcerated. Intravascular diffuse large B-cell lymphoma is a proliferation of large B-cells within blood vessels, but in some cases, the skin can be the only affected site. The cutaneous findings in this subtype include indurated, erythematous or violaceous patches or plaques that tend to occur on the trunk and thighs.

ii. There are no specific laboratory value abnormalities that are routinely found associated with primary cutaneous B-cell lymphomas. Of note, lactose dehydrogenase (LDH) levels should be normal, in contrast to elevated LDH levels in systemic lymphomas. Additional work-up must be performed to complete staging of each case of pCBCL, which should include complete blood count, flow cytometry of peripheral blood and computed tomography (CT) imaging of the chest, abdomen and pelvis. Bone marrow biopsy with flow cytometry of the aspirate is recommended in follicle centre lymphoma.

iii. In primary cutaneous follicle centre lymphoma, there are diffuse or nodular infiltrates throughout the dermis and subcutaneous fat. A follicular pattern with formation of neoplastic germinal centres is seen in approximately 25% of cases. The infiltrate is composed of centroblasts and centrocytes admixed with immunoblasts, small lymphocytes and occasionally plasma cells and histiocytes.

iv. Primary cutaneous follicle centre lymphoma is indolent with a favourable prognosis. Recurrence is reported in up to 50% of cases but dissemination to lymph nodes or internal organs is exceedingly rare. Many patients with low-grade pCBCL can be managed conservatively with follow-up examinations every 6 months. Skin lesions can be treated locally with intralesional corticosteroids, local radiotherapy or surgical excision. There are a few reports of successful treatment of low-grade pCBCL with systemic antibiotics, intralesional interferon-α-2a and rituximab.

CASE 57

Cutaneous T-cell lymphoma

QUESTION 57

A 58-year-old African American man presents as a referral for the evaluation of a patchy, erythematous, pruritic rash that is primarily on his trunk and legs. The rash has been present for about 20 years and has expanded progressively from initially involving his lower back and buttock to spreading to his legs and upper back. Previous biopsies have been performed, which showed a possible contact dermatitis. He was also treated with numerous antifungal shampoos and creams, but showed no improvement. On examination, there are numerous eczematous erythematous patches and plaques on the back, chest, arms and legs, involving approximately 75% of the patient's total body surface area (57a, b).

57a

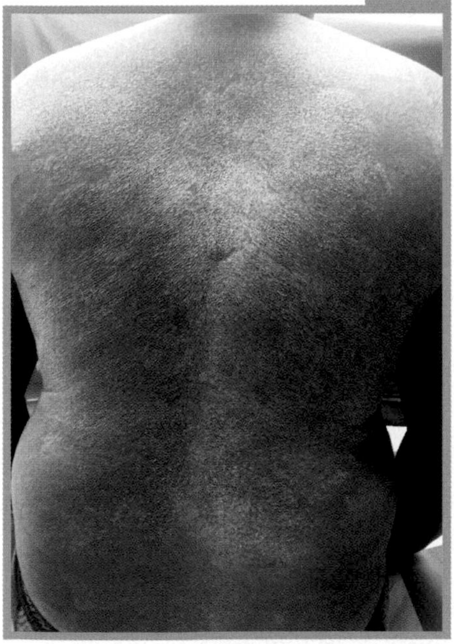

57b

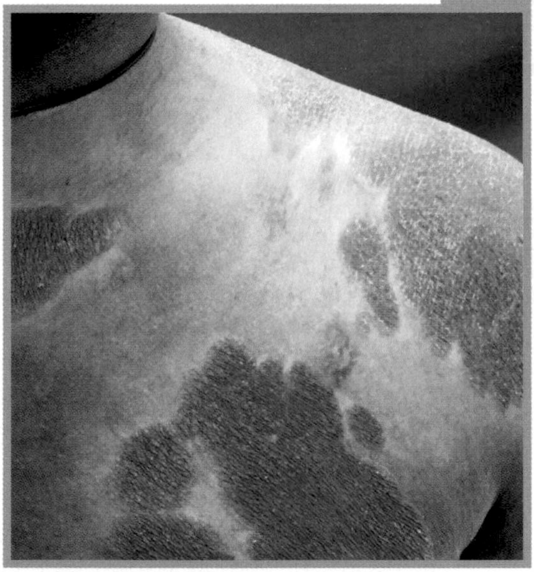

i. This patient's disease most likely falls within what group of conditions?

ii. What are the histopathologic findings of this disease, and what additional testing can lead to a specific diagnosis?

iii. What are the treatment options?

Answer 57

i. This patient has cutaneous T-cell lymphoma (CTCL), which describes a group of neoplasms of skin-homing T cells. CTCL accounts for 75%–80% of all primary cutaneous lymphomas, whereas primary B-cell lymphomas account for 20%–25%. There are several types of CTCLs that have been defined based on clinical, histological and immunophenotypical criteria. These entities can vary considerably in both their clinical presentation and disease course.

The clinical presentation of this patient is consistent with classical mycosis fungoides (MF). The course is often indolent, extending over years. Many patients experience several years of nonspecific eczematous and psoriasiform skin findings and non-diagnostic skin biopsies. The median time from the development of skin lesions to the diagnosis of mycosis fungoides is 4–6 years. In the classical type, the early patch stage is characterized by variably-sized, erythematous, hyperpigmented patches that often involve the buttocks and other covered sites of the trunk and limbs. Progression can lead to infiltrated red-brown plaques (plaque stage MF) and in some patients, nodules and tumours (tumour stage MF).

There are other clinical variants of MF, including folliculotropic MF, hypopigmented MF, pagetoid reticulosis (also known as Woringer–Kolopp disease) and granulomatous slack skin, among others.

ii. Histologically, MF is characterized by a lymphocytic lichenoid infiltrate containing atypical cells with small- to medium-sized cerebriform nuclei confined to the epidermis. In early patch stage lesions, the epidermotropism may be subtle, becoming more pronounced in the plaque stage of MF. Intraepidermal nests of atypical cells, known as Pautrier's microabscesses are characteristic features of MF but are only observed in a minority of cases. With progression to the tumour stage, dermal infiltrates are more evident and may extend down to the subcutaneous tissue.

Immunophenotyping can occasionally provide additional information. The neoplastic cells of MF have a CD8-memory T-cell phenotype, which is positive for CD3 and CD4. However, aberrant phenotypes are typically observed in plaque or tumour stage MF and rarely assist in the diagnosis of early patch stage MF.

iii. The therapeutic approach to MF is dependent on both the stage of the disease and the age and condition of the patient. Skin-directed therapies are preferred in early stages of MF (IA–IIA) or limited tumour stage MF (IIB). These include topical or intralesional corticosteroids, topical chemotherapy (mechlorethamine, carmustine), radiotherapy or phototherapy. Systemic therapy is considered in patients with refractory or progressive skin disease. Some agents that are used in combination are oral retinoids (isotretinoin, etretinate, acitretin, bexarotene), interferon alpha, denileukin diftitox and histone deacetylase inhibitors such as vorinostat and depsipeptide. Systemic treatment is usually a multi-agent chemotherapy, and the most common regimen used is cyclophosphamide, hydroxydaunomycin, vincristine and prednisone. This is reserved only for patients with lymph node or visceral involvement or in patients with progressive skin tumours recalcitrant to prior treatments.

CASE 58

Leukemia cutis

QUESTION 58

A 68-year-old man presents to his general practitioner with a 9-month history of progressive fatigue, nausea and rash. He has noticed increased fatigue with minimal exertion, which has prevented him from performing his usual activities. He also states that he initially noticed red bumps on his shoulders, which are asymptomatic but continue to spread across his chest and back. On examination, there are scattered erythematous to violaceous papules and nodules, some coalescing into plaques distributed over the chest, back, arms and face (58a, b). Laboratory studies reveal a marked lymphocytosis (white blood cells [WBC] 46 × 10^9/L) and a peripheral smear is composed of >25% blasts and 'smudge' cells.

58a

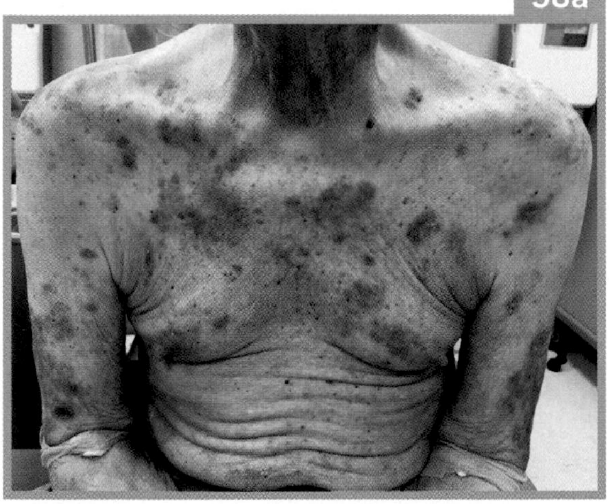

58b

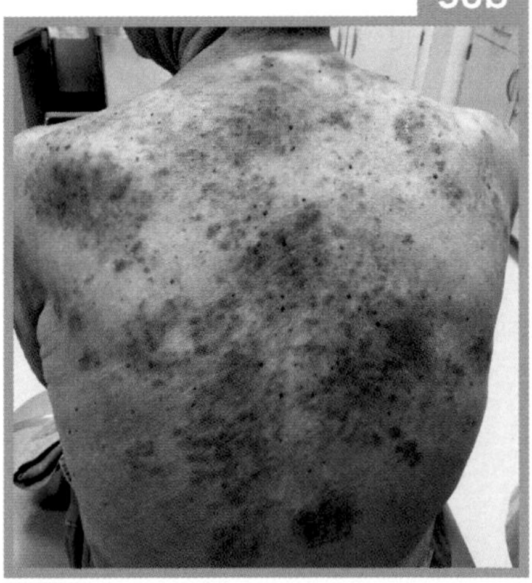

i. What is the cause of his rash?

ii. What are the other conditions that can be seen in the setting of this patient's disease?

iii. What features are seen on the histopathologic examination, and what immunohistochemical stains will confirm the diagnosis?

Answer 58

i. The patient presents with chronic lymphocytic leukemia (CLL), which is supported by his laboratory reports and peripheral blood smear. His rash is consistent with leukemia cutis, which represents dermal infiltrates of neoplastic cells. Leukemia cutis can occur anywhere on the body but most often involves the head, neck and trunk or demonstrates a predilection for sites of trauma or scars. They typically present as firm papules and nodules that can be hemorrhagic and rarely ulcerative. They are often asymptomatic and can be the presenting sign leading to the diagnosis of leukemia.

ii. Leukemia cutis accounts for up to 30% of cutaneous biopsies in patients with leukemia. Other cutaneous findings that are associated with leukemia include Sweet's syndrome, pyoderma gangrenosum, neutrophilic eccrine hidradenitis, erythroderma, and erythema nodosum, among others.

iii. Leukemia cutis can demonstrate a wide range of histologic features, but a common finding is a dense neoplastic infiltrate that can be perivascular, nodular or diffuse. The neoplastic infiltrate will display atypical features with immature lymphocytes that aid in diagnosis. In CLL, immunohistochemistry will be positive for CD5, CD20 and CD43 antigens.

CASE 59

Kaposi sarcoma

QUESTION 59

A 27-year-old man with a history notable for human immunodeficiency virus/acquired immunodeficiency syndrome (HIV/AIDS) presents to the dermatology clinic for the evaluation of a new rash on his chest. The lesions have been present for 1–2 months and have progressively spread over his body. They are painless and do not bother him otherwise. His past medical history is significant for HIV with AIDS-defining illnesses including pneumocystis pneumonia and cryptococcal meningitis due to poor adherence to antiretroviral therapy. On examination, there are scattered violaceous macules, papules and nodules on the chest (59a). Upon inspection of the oral mucosa, there is a violaceous plaque on the hard palate with areas of ulceration (59b). Review of recent laboratory studies reveals a CD4 count of 40 cells/mm^3 and a viral load of 475,000 copies/mL.

59a

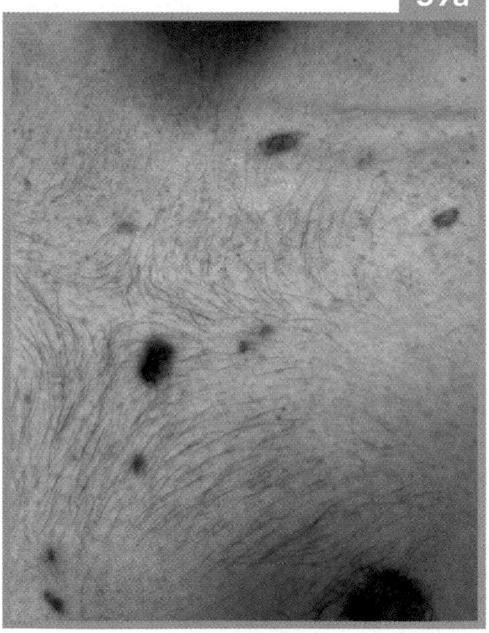

59b

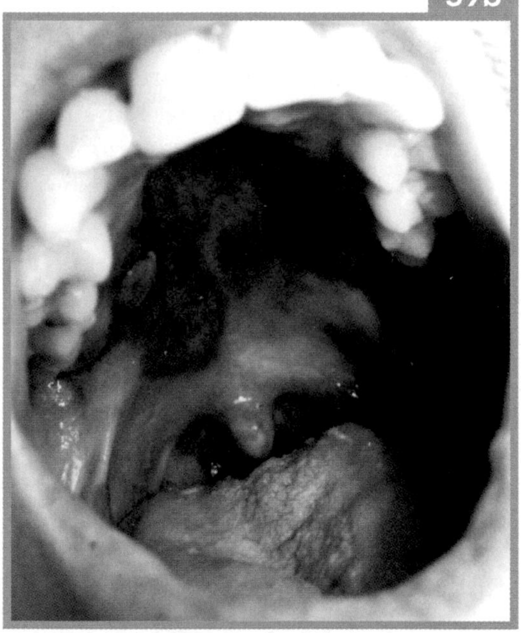

i. What is the diagnosis?

ii. What are the four types of this disease?

iii. What are the characteristic histopathologic and immunohistochemical findings?

Answer 59

i. This patient with AIDS presents with Kaposi sarcoma (KS), which is an endothelial malignancy. Initially described in elderly men of Ashkenazi Jewish or Mediterranean descent, Kaposi sarcoma became more widely known as it became increasingly reported among young men with AIDS in the 1980s. Kaposi sarcoma is associated with human herpesvirus-8 (HHV-8) in the vast majority of cases, although there are different hypotheses regarding the exact role of HHV-8 in the pathogenesis of KS.

ii. There are four different types of KS, which include: (1) classic KS, (2) AIDS-related KS, (3) immunosuppression-related KS and (4) African-endemic KS. The different types of KS vary in their clinical presentation and disease course. Classic KS is characterized by the development of violaceous plaques, primarily found on the legs of elderly men of Mediterranean descent. In its classic form, KS rarely involves the oral mucosa or gastrointestinal tract and has an indolent clinical course. In AIDS-related KS, patients often present with a wide distribution of erythematous-to-violaceous papules or plaques that tend to affect the oral cavity, face, genital mucosa and gastrointestinal tract more often than classic KS, with up to 80% of AIDS patients developing gastrointestinal involvement. The clinical course of AIDS-related KS is variable, largely dependent on the degree of immune compromise. Immunosuppression-associated KS is seen in patients on immunosuppressive medications and shares many clinical features with AIDS-related KS. African-endemic KS can present as nodular, lymphoadenopathic,

59c

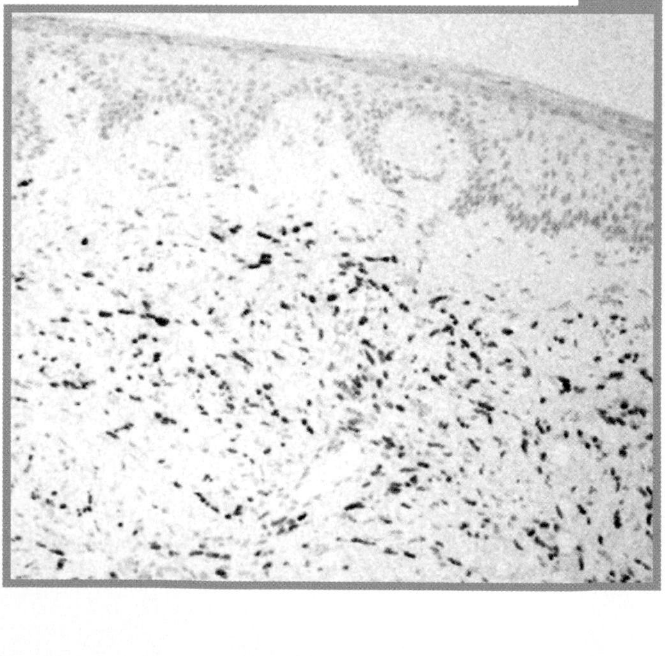

florid or infiltrative disease. Nodular African-endemic KS typically follows an indolent course, whereas the lymphadenopathic, florid and infiltrative forms can be aggressive and fatal.

iii. Skin biopsies can be performed to confirm the diagnosis of KS. Histologically, all types of KS are characterized by the proliferation of spindle-shaped cells surrounding vascular channels with atypical endothelial cells. Perivascular lymphocytic infiltrates are commonly seen. Immunohistochemical staining against latent nuclear antigen-1 will demonstrate the presence of HHV-8 (59c).

CASE 60

Angiosarcoma

QUESTION 60

A 75-year-old woman is evaluated by the dermatology inpatient consult service for an enlarging growth on her forehead. She states that this area initially started as a small bruise on the right forehead, but rapidly progressed with swelling and the appearance of violaceous, hemorrhagic plaques and nodules with ulceration (60). She also states that it is very itchy and painful. Biopsy revealed infiltration of the dermis by vascular spaces lined by piled-up endothelial cells splitting apart collagen bundles.

60

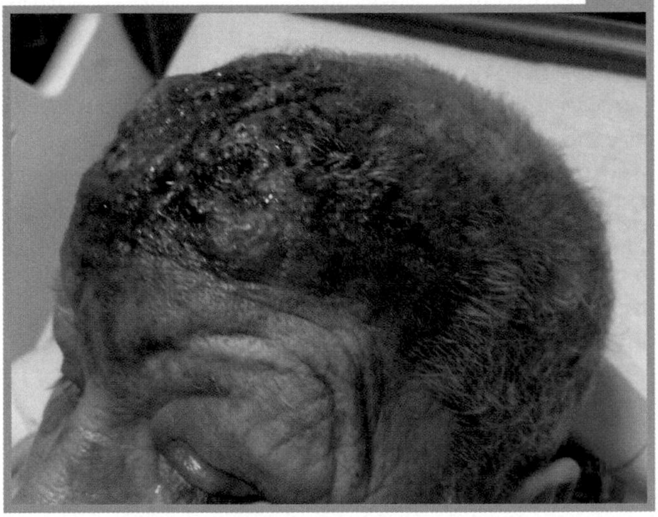

i. What is the diagnosis?

ii. What is the treatment of choice and overall prognosis for this condition?

iii. This same histologic diagnosis can also arise in the setting of chronic lymphedema post-mastectomy. What is that syndrome called?

Answer 60

i. This patient has cutaneous angiosarcoma, which is an uncommon high-grade malignant neoplasm of endothelial derivation and accounts for <1% of all sarcomas. Angiosarcoma has a predilection for skin and superficial soft tissue, and most commonly arises on the scalp and face of the elderly or in the setting of chronic lymphedema or radiodermatitis. A highly variable degree of endothelial differentiation can be seen in cutaneous angiosarcomas.

ii. The treatment of choice is surgical excision with wide margins. Even with negative margins, the risk of recurrence and metastatic disease is high. Prognosis is poor with a 5-year survival rate of <15%.

iii. Angiosarcoma associated with chronic lymphedema typically presents as firm violaceous plaques or nodules in an area of non-pitting edema. The most common area of involvement is the upper arm, associated with lymphedema in patients with a history of breast cancer treated with mastectomy and lymph node dissection. This association, known as Stewart–Treves syndrome, makes up more than 90% of all angiosarcomas associated with lymphedema. Although the reported incidence of angiosarcoma in breast cancer survivors is very low (<0.05%), an increase in postirradiation sarcomas has been observed, likely in part due to improved treatment options with an emphasis on breast-sparing surgeries such as lumpectomy over radical mastectomy.

INFECTIONS

CASE 61

Scabies

QUESTION 61

A 41-year-old man with a remote history of Hodgkin's lymphoma presents with an intensely pruritic rash that is scattered over his arms and legs and in his groin region. He states that the eruption began on his wrists and hands and has progressively spread. He denies any history of atopic dermatitis or recent travel. A skin scraping was performed with a scalpel blade and was observed under the light microscope using mineral oil (61).

61

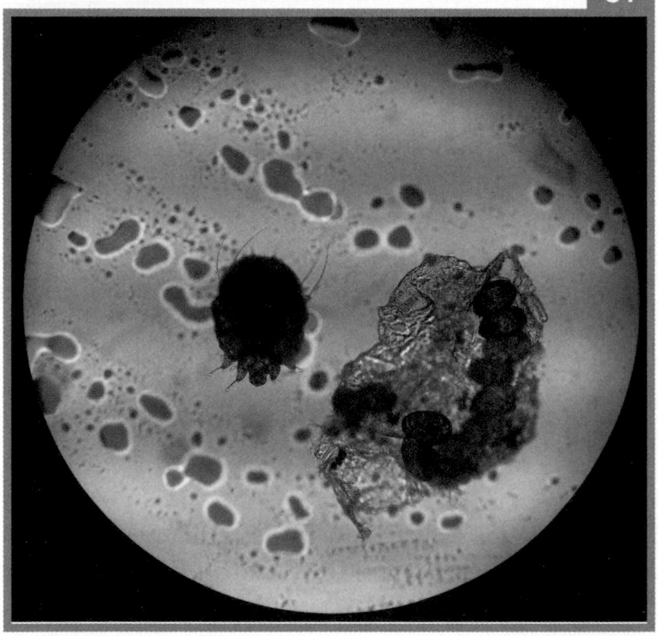

i. What does Figure 61 show?

ii. What is the most appropriate treatment for this patient and his family?

iii. What is a more severe variant of this disease and in which two special populations is it more likely to be found?

Answer 61

i. Figure 61 shows a scabies mite, known as *Sarcoptes scabiei* var. *hominus*, along with several eggs. Scabies mites are human host-specific, and live their entire 30-day life cycle within the epidermis. Too small to be seen by the naked eye, mites lay eggs that mature over 10 days. The incubation period of scabies infestation is 2–6 weeks, depending on the host's immune system. A second infestation can manifest within 24–48 hours. Cutaneous manifestations of scabies are typically small, erythematous papules or vesicles with associated burrows, which are pathognomonic for scabies. The burrow is a thread-like wavy tunnel created by a female mite while laying eggs. The most common sites of burrows are the interdigital webbing of the hands, wrists, axillae and groin. In infants and the elderly, all skin surfaces can be involved, including the scalp and face. Patients presenting with scabies infestations characteristically experience extreme pruritus with worse pruritus reported at night. Secondary bacterial infections with *Streptococcus pyogenes* or *S. aureus* can develop.

ii. Scabies infestation is transmitted by direct or close contact with an infested person. Less commonly, fomite transmission is possible but is usually only seen in severe cases. Treatment involves two topical scabicidal applications, 1 week apart. The most common topical treatments are permethrin 5% cream, a synthetic pyrethroid that paralyzes arthropods, and lindane 1% lotion or cream, an organochlorine agent. Due to the potential neurotoxic side effects associated with lindane, it is contraindicated in infants, individuals with crusted scabies, seizure disorders or other underlying skin conditions that can increase systemic absorption, such as atopic dermatitis. It should be used with caution in children, the elderly and other individuals weighing less than 50 kg. Topical treatment involves application to the entire affected body surface overnight. At the time of each treatment, clothing, linens and towels should be washed with hot water and dried with high heat to reduce the risk of reinfestation. Oral ivermectin is an off-label treatment that can be used to treat scabies. Because of the relatively high rate of asymptomatic mite carriers in households, all family members and close contacts should undergo treatment, even if asymptomatic.

iii. Crusted scabies is a severe variant of scabies, in which patients can have infestations of thousands of mites on the skin surface, in comparison to typical scabies infections in which there are less than a hundred mites. Due to the higher volume of mites, this form of scabies is highly contagious and transmission through fomites is more common. The scabies mites in crusted scabies can also live longer (up to 7 days) by feeding on sloughed skin. Clinically, crusted scabies presents as marked hyperkeratosis that can be widespread but tends to favour acral sites. Pruritus is typically less prominent. It can be seen more in two special populations: (1) immunocompromised hosts, such as the elderly, solid organ transplant recipients and patients with human immunodeficiency virus (HIV) and (2) patients with decreased sensation or ability to scratch, such as patients with leprosy or paraplegia.

CASE 62

Bullous impetigo

QUESTION 62

A 12-year-old Hispanic girl presents with an 8-day history of recurrent blisters on both legs. She initially thought that it was due to a mosquito bite but became concerned when she began to develop larger blisters, some of which appeared pus-filled. On examination, there were round excoriated plaques with a collarette of scale. There was one intact blister filled with clear and purulent fluid (62a, b). A skin biopsy demonstrates a subcorneal blister with an inflammatory infiltrate in the dermis consisting of neutrophils. Gram-positive cocci can be seen in the superficial epidermis.

62a

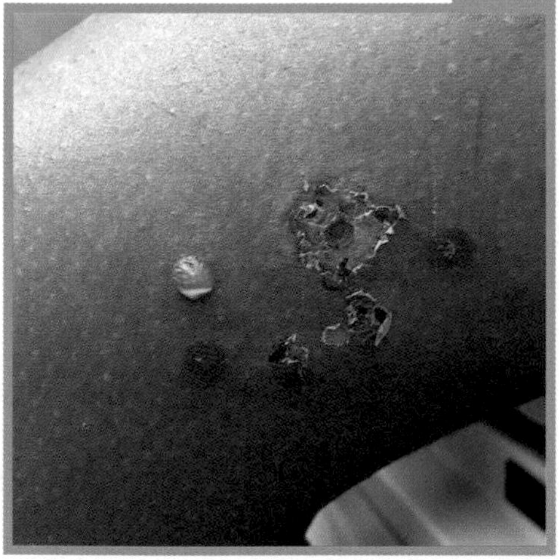

62b

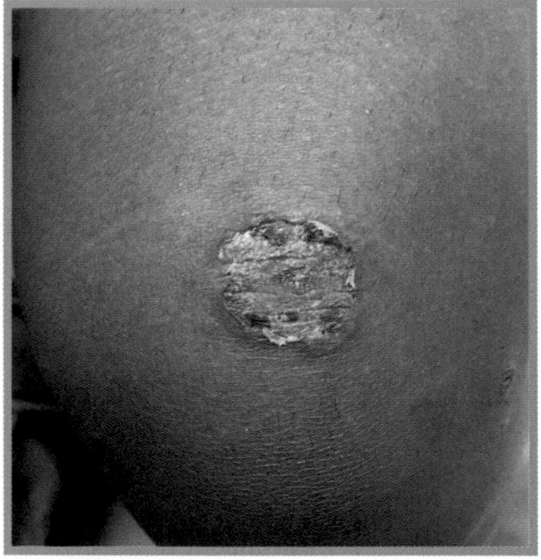

i. What is the diagnosis? What is/are the most common causative agent(s)?

ii. What populations are most often affected?

iii. What complications can be seen and what is the treatment?

Answer 62

i. The clinical and histopathologic presentation is consistent with bullous impetigo, a bullous form of a superficial cutaneous infection most commonly due to *Staphylococcus aureus*. Non-bullous impetigo, which is more common, is due to *S. aureus* and *Streptococcus pyogenes*.

Bullous impetigo is characterized by small vesicles that enlarge into flaccid bullae that rupture and leave behind a collarette of scale. There is typically minimal surrounding erythema and no systemic symptoms, although some patients may have associated fever and weakness.

ii. Bullous impetigo is most often seen in neonates, but may also be seen in children and adolescents as well as immunocompromised patients or patients with chronic renal disease. In these patients, the exfoliative toxin can become disseminated and lead to the development of staphylococcal scalded skin syndrome.

iii. In about 5% of cases, non-bullous impetigo caused by *S. pyogenes* can be complicated by acute post-streptococcal glomerulonephritis.

Uncomplicated bullous impetigo is self-limited and resolves without scarring in 3–6 weeks. Topical antibiotics such as mupirocin appear to be as efficacious as systemic antibiotics in limited cutaneous disease. For complicated impetigo, first-line therapy is ceftriaxone by intravenous (IV) administration, and second-line therapy is ampicillin/sulbactam or cefuroxime.

CASE 63

Syphilis

QUESTION 63

A 42-year-old man presents to the dermatology clinic with a 2-week history of a spreading rash. He states that the rash began on his chest and abdomen and spread to his arms, legs, as well as his palms and soles. The rash is completely asymptomatic. He denies any recent illnesses or sick contacts, but he recalls an episode of a penile ulcer approximately 2 months ago, which resolved without any intervention. On examination, there is a generalized light pink papular rash on the back, chest and abdomen (63a). On the hands, there are red-brown macules scattered on the palmar aspects of the hands and fingers (63b).

63a

63b

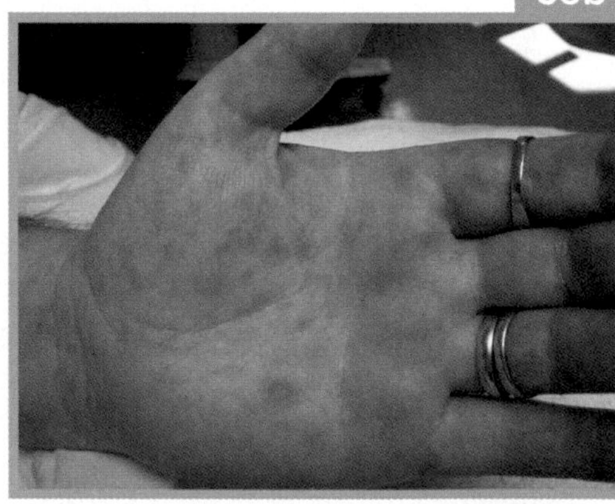

i. What is the diagnosis and causative pathogen? What tests can be performed to confirm the diagnosis?

ii. What is the time course of the different stages of this infection? What are the cutaneous findings associated with each stage?

iii. What complication can be observed with treatment?

Answer 63

i. The patient presents with a history and clinical findings consistent with secondary syphilis, a sexually transmitted infection caused by the spirochete, *Treponema pallidum*. Serological tests can be performed to help confirm the diagnosis. The non-treponemal tests include Venereal Disease Research Laboratory (VDRL) and rapid plasma reagin (RPR), which become reactive 4–5 weeks after infection and revert to non-reactive states during latent stages of the disease and after treatment. Although these tests demonstrate high sensitivity, conditions such as pregnancy, other spirochete infections, certain viral infections (human immunodeficiency virus [HIV], infectious mononucleosis) and autoimmune diseases such as systemic lupus erythematosus can lead to falsely positive non-treponemal tests. Treponemal tests include fluorescent treponemal antibody absorption (FTA-ABS) and microhemagglutination assay for *T. pallidum* (MHA-TP). FTA-ABS is positive by 3 weeks after infection and remains positive after treatment, whereas MHA-TP is less sensitive during primary syphilis. ELISA demonstrates 100% specificity and is useful during early or congenital infection, but is less sensitive in later stages of disease. Dark-field microscopy can also be performed to confirm the diagnosis, however, it is not widely available.

ii. After inoculation, the primary stage of syphilis occurs after an incubation period of 10–90 days (average 3 weeks). The secondary stage of syphilis occurs 3–10 weeks after the appearance of primary syphilis in almost all untreated patients. It represents the hematogenous and lymphatic dissemination of treponemes in different tissues and thus demonstrates a wide spectrum of clinical manifestations. Following secondary syphilis, a period of latency can occur and last for many years. Approximately 70% of patients enter a period of latency and remain immune to new primary infections. Latent syphilis is divided into early and late latency periods. The remainder of individuals may progress to the tertiary stage or late stage of syphilis, in which the microorganism invades the central nervous and cardiovascular systems.

Clinically, primary syphilis manifests as a firm, well-circumscribed, painless chancre arising on mucosal surfaces such as the mouth, genitals or anus, with or without associated lymphadenopathy. These may go unnoticed when they occur inside the vagina or anus. In the secondary stage, prodromal symptoms such as low-grade fever, malaise, conjunctivitis, pharyngitis, adenopathy and weight loss are frequently reported. In the skin, secondary syphilis presents as a generalized non-pruritic eruption that can range in colour from pink to red-brown. It usually occurs on the trunk and affects the palms and soles. Infiltrations of treponemes manifest as condylomata lata in the anogenital region and as corona veneris along the hairline. On the mucous membranes, mucous patches and syphilitic perleche can be observed. Less commonly, secondary syphilis can manifest as patchy alopecia with a characteristic 'moth-eaten' appearance. Tertiary syphilis is characterized by the development of gummas or locally destructive lesions in the organs. In the skin, gummas present as nodular or noduloulcerative lesions that involute over weeks to months with residual scarring. Tertiary syphilis can also affect the central nervous system (CNS) and cardiovascular system, leading to neurosyphilis and aortitis, respectively.

iii. The treatment of choice for all stages of syphilis is penicillin G. A Jarisch–Herxheimer reaction can be observed upon treatment of early syphilis, which is caused by the release of inflammatory cytokines such as tumour necrosis factor-alpha (TNF-α) due to phagocytosis of the spirochetes after antibiotic administration. It is characterized by fever, headache, lymphadenopathy, myalgias and leukocytosis. It can be managed with supportive care and should not lead to cessation of treatment.

CASE 64

Erythema migrans

QUESTION 64

A 21-year-old otherwise healthy man presents to the dermatology clinic with an enlarging rash on the trunk. He works as a landscaper and states that no one else at work has a similar-appearing rash. The patient reports noticing the lesion on his upper trunk approximately 4 days ago when he also experienced fatigue, a low-grade fever, and chills. On examination, there are two expanding erythematous-to-violaceous plaques on the left lateral trunk with central clearing and a brightly erythematous border (64).

64

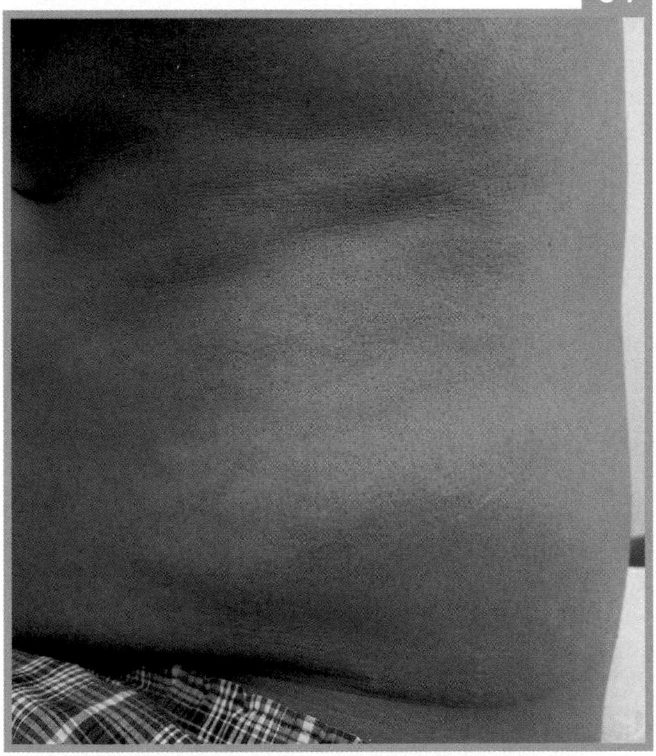

i. What are these lesions called, and what is the aetiology?

ii. What diagnostic tests can be performed, and what are their limitations?

iii. What is the cutaneous finding of this disease in its chronic form?

iv. What are the treatment options?

Answer 64

i. Lyme disease is a tick-borne, multisystem disease that is caused by infection with *Borrelia* species of spirochetes. In the United States, most cases of Lyme disease are caused by *Borrelia burgdorferi*, whereas *B. garinii* and *B. afzelii* are the predominant etiologic organisms seen in Europe. The *Ixodes* tick acts as the vector for disease transmission by feeding on an infected host (usually white-footed mice and white-tailed deer) and transmitting the bacteria to humans through its saliva.

The patient's lesions are a classic cutaneous manifestation of early-localized Lyme disease, called erythema migrans. It is an annular erythematous rash with central clearing or a bull's-eye appearance that develops at the site of the tick bite within 1–2 weeks. Systemic manifestations of early Lyme disease are flu-like symptoms such as fever, fatigue, arthralgias, myalgias and lymphadenopathy. In up to 25% of patients there may be numerous lesions of erythema migrans which occur as a result of multiple tick bites, or in disseminated disease due to lymphatic spread or spirochetemia. In chronic Lyme disease, patients develop monoarticular or oligoarticular arthritis, neurological manifestations such as Bell's palsy and/or cardiac complications such as atrioventricular block.

ii. The diagnosis of Lyme disease does not require a history of tick bite. Testing can be performed with the enzyme-linked immunosorbent assay (ELISA) or Western blot analysis, but antibodies often remain for months or years after infection, and therefore cannot distinguish between active and past infection. Skin biopsy and culture can also be performed but is not routinely done. Histologically, the presence of an infiltrate composed of eosinophils and plasma cells within the dermis supports the diagnosis, but is not a specific finding to erythema migrans.

iii. Acrodermatitis chronica atrophicans (ACA), also known as Herxheimer disease, is a cutaneous manifestation of chronic Lyme disease. It is most commonly associated with Lyme disease through infection with *B. afzelii,* and therefore seen in higher frequency (up to 10%) in people with Lyme disease in Europe than in the United States. It is characterized by an initial presentation of erythematous and violaceous nodules and plaques on acral surfaces, any time between 6 months and 8 years after infection. In the late stage of ACA, the skin becomes atrophic, shiny and wrinkled, with prominent blood vessels. It can also lead to dyspigmentation, pain and pruritus.

iv. Treatment of Lyme disease includes early removal of the tick, and initiation of antibiotics. In early localized or mild disseminated disease, the first-line therapy is doxycycline for 2–4 weeks of therapy. Children and pregnant women should be treated with amoxicillin as an alternative agent. In severe disseminated disease or chronic Lyme disease with significant neurologic or cardiac complications, first-line therapy is intravenous ceftriaxone for 2–4 weeks.

CASE 65

Lepromatous leprosy

QUESTION 65

A 22-year-old man who recently emigrated from Brazil presents to the dermatology clinic with a generalized rash on his face, back and extremities. He also reports symptoms of fever, myalgias and left knee swelling. He worked as an industrial painter but has found it increasingly difficult to hold on to paint brushes due to diminished sensation in his hands. On examination, there are innumerable, red to violaceous infiltrated nodules distributed on his ears, back and legs (65a–c).

65a

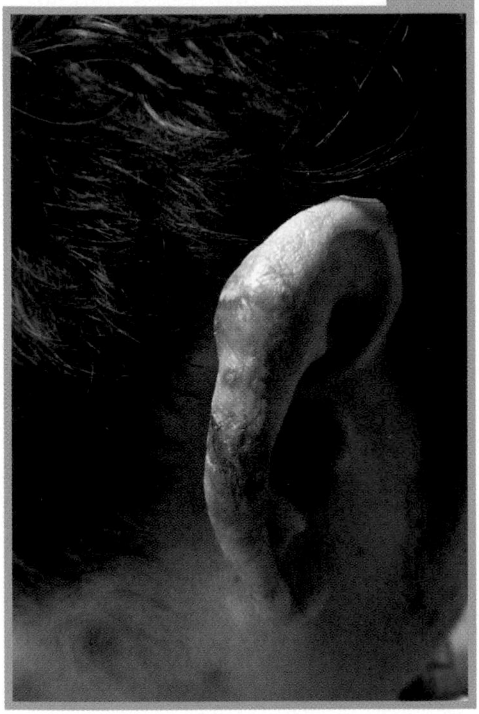

65b

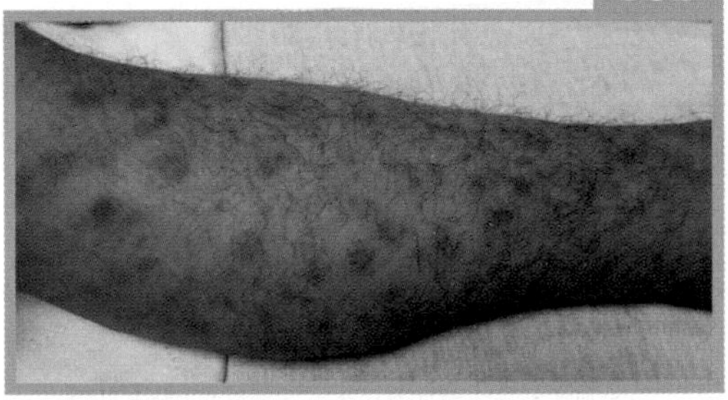

65c

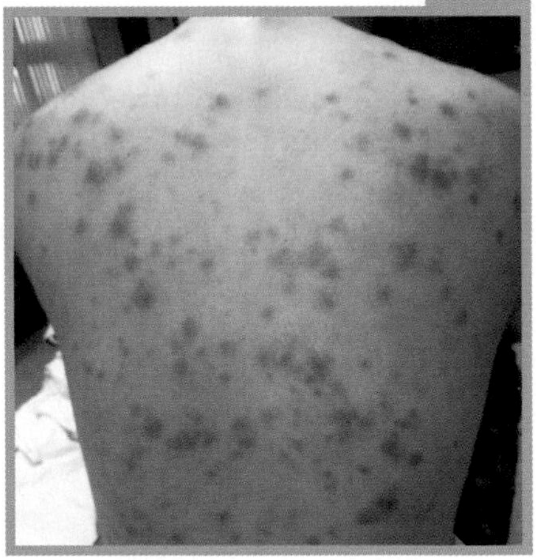

i. What is the diagnosis?

ii. What type of reaction is this, and what are other commonly associated systemic symptoms?

iii. What is the treatment of choice?

Answer 65

i. This patient has lepromatous leprosy, a chronic infectious disease caused by *Mycobacterium leprae*, an acid fast bacillus. Though there is a wide spectrum of clinical findings in leprosy, this patient demonstrates skin lesions characteristic of erythema nodosum leprosum, which is typically seen in lepromatous leprosy.

ii. There are two major types of lepromatous reactional states. Type 1 is a delayed-type hypersensitivity reaction that is seen in borderline or tuberculoid leprosy and often occurs during or after treatment. This patient is presenting with a type 2 reactional state, which is due to the formation of immune complexes and results in cutaneous and systemic small vessel vasculitis. The most common clinical manifestation is erythema nodosum leprosum. It is seen more commonly in lepromatous leprosy, particularly among patients with a high bacterial index who are undergoing treatment. Along with characteristic nodular skin lesions, patients can experience fever, myalgias, malaise, severe joint swelling and pain, iridocyclitis, lymphadenitis, hepatosplenomegaly, orchitis and glomerulonephritis.

iii. For the treatment of leprosy, the World Health Organization recommends multidrug regimens. In patients with paucibacillary leprosy, treatment includes rifampin monthly with a sulfone such as dapsone daily for 6 months, then observation for 2 years. For patients with at least one bacillus detected via bacilloscopy, treatment includes rifampin, clofazimine and dapsone for 1–2 years, then observation for 5 years. In patients with evidence of either of the two major inflammatory reactions, additional treatment is typically required. For type 1 reactions, the treatment of choice is oral prednisone. For type 2 reactions, the treatment of choice is thalidomide. Additional drugs that may benefit type 2 reactions include clofazimine, cyclosporine, chloroquine, pentoxifylline and phosphodiesterase type-4 inhibitors such as roflumilast.

CASE 66

Atypical mycobacteria

QUESTION 66

A 34-year-old man presents to the emergency department with fever, chills and a 5-day history of progressive swelling and pain in his right lower extremity. He is on chronic immunosuppression due to a deceased-donor kidney transplant. He does not recall any inciting trauma to the area. He states that he recently took his children to a water park several weeks ago. On examination, the distal foot is erythematous and with notable edema as well as suppurative abscesses scattered on the foot and tracking up in a lymphocutaneous distribution (66).

66

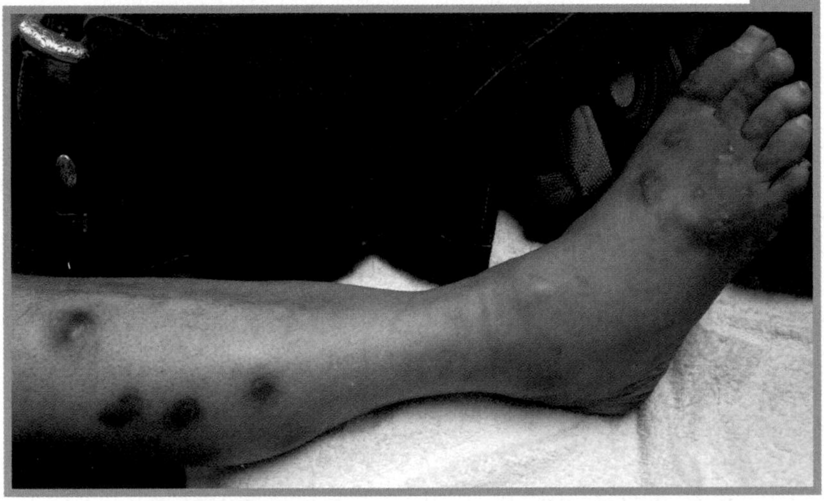

i. What is the most likely aetiology of these findings?

ii. How can the diagnosis be confirmed?

iii. What is the first step in management?

Answer 66

i. Given this patient's co-morbidities, his presentation is most consistent with an atypical mycobacterial infection, which is caused by nontuberculous mycobacteria. These are organisms found in the environment in water, wet soil, house dust, dairy products, vegetation and human feces. Transmission occurs through inhalation, ingestion or percutaneous penetration. Depending on the causative organism, clinical presentation can range from pustules, keratotic plaques, nodules or ulcers with draining sinuses. In immunosuppressed individuals, disseminated infections can occur.

With a reported history of swimming pool exposure, the causative agent in this patient is likely *Mycobacterium marinum*, also known as fish tank granuloma or swimming pool granuloma. This organism is one of the most commonly identified species in nontuberculous mycobacterial skin infections. It is found in fresh, salt and brackish water, but can also be found in swimming pools as it is relatively resistant to chlorine. After absorption by a portal of entry (usually percutaneous via incidental trauma), the incubation period lasts for 3–4 weeks. The initial lesion occurs at the portal of entry and forms a crusted ulcer, suppurative abscess or nodule, followed by the development of additional nodules along the draining lymphatics. Infection with *M. marinum* can be complicated by tenosynovitis, septic arthritis or rarely osteomyelitis.

ii. The diagnosis can be confirmed by obtaining cultures. *Mycobacterium marinum* grows best at 31°C, and when grown at optimal temperatures, the yield of cultures can be as high as 70%–80%.

iii. As this patient demonstrates signs of systemic involvement (fever, chills), ensuring hemodynamic stability is a priority. Although definitive antimicrobial therapy will depend on the causative organism, empiric treatment with clarithromycin while awaiting culture results can be considered in this patient with a cutaneous nontuberculous mycobacterial infection. Once the diagnosis is confirmed by culture, *M. marinum* can be treated with clarithromycin, minocycline, doxycycline, rifampin, ethambutol or trimethoprim–sulfamethoxazole. In patients with disseminated disease, treatment with at least two agents is preferred.

CASE 67

Herpes zoster

QUESTION 67

A 75-year-old man with a history of chronic obstructive pulmonary disease (COPD) and colon cancer presents with a 3-day history of an intensely pruritic and painful rash on his left mid-back. He states that it began as a tingling area before he began to develop multiple blisters. He does not have any other sites of involvement. On examination, there is a unilateral erythematous rash consisting of papules and vesicles in a dermatomal distribution on the back (67a).

67a

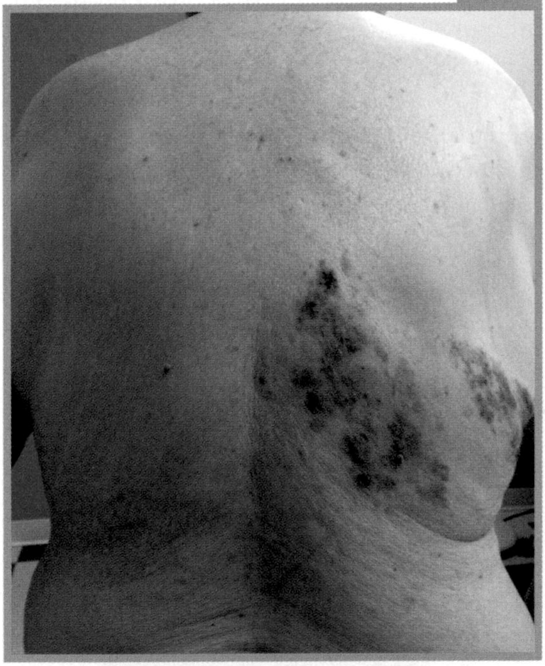

i. Which human herpesvirus is responsible for this eruption?

ii. What is the clinical sign suggestive of ocular involvement?

iii. What is the syndrome that can lead to facial nerve paralysis?

iv. What underlying disease should be considered in multidermatomal, verrucous or disseminated presentations?

v. What is the treatment of choice, and what are the common sequelae of this disease?

Answer 67

i. This patient presents with shingles, also known as herpes zoster, which is a reactivation of varicella-zoster virus or human herpesvirus-3. Herpes zoster often presents first with a prodrome of pruritus, pain or tingling in the dermatome involved, followed by the development of painful grouped vesicles in a dermatomal distribution. Occasionally, vesicles can involve more than one contiguous dermatome and cross the midline. The most common sites affected are the trunk and face.

ii. 'Hutchinson's sign' is the presence of skin lesions in the distribution of the nasociliary branch of nerves, which supplies the nasal tip, dorsum and root of the nose. This is seen with infection of the ophthalmic division of the trigeminal nerve, which is seen in 10%–15% of patients with herpes zoster. It is important to recognize ocular involvement, because ocular scarring and visual loss are potential sequelae.

iii. Ramsay Hunt syndrome is a herpes zoster infection of the geniculate ganglion. In this syndrome, herpes zoster involves the external ear and face and can lead to tinnitus or other auditory symptoms, as well as ipsilateral facial paralysis (67b).

67b

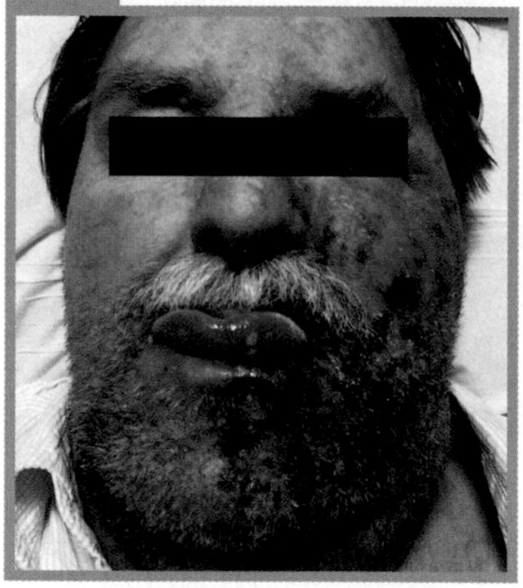

iv. In patients with human immunodeficiency virus (HIV), herpes zoster can manifest with unusual presentations, which include multidermatomal, verrucous and disseminated. Disseminated herpes zoster, defined as the presence of more than 20 vesicles outside of the area of primary dermatomal involvement or adjacent dermatomes, should lead clinicians to also consider visceral involvement, most commonly hepatic, pulmonary and central nervous system (CNS) infection. Patients who present with these variants should be tested for HIV.

v. Food and Drug Administration (FDA)-approved treatments for herpes zoster include acyclovir, famciclovir and valacyclovir. Treatment should be initiated within 72 hours of the development of skin lesions, although benefit is seen with initiation within 7 days. Treatment with antiviral medication also reduces the frequency and duration of common sequelae such as postherpetic neuralgia. Although most cases of herpes zoster resolve without sequelae in children and young adults, postherpetic neuralgia is a common complication in older patients or patients with immune compromise. Treatment for postherpetic neuralgia includes low-dose tricyclic antidepressants, gabapentin, topical capsaicin, transepidermal nerve stimulation, local analgesics and nerve blocks.

CASE 68

Candidiasis

QUESTION 68

A 78-year-old man with a history of prostate cancer and osteoarthritis presents with a 3-month history of a burning, tender rash in the groin. He reports that it worsened over the last several months after he suffered a fall and was immobilized in bed for several weeks. He has tried to treat the area with numerous over-the-counter antifungals, which helps reduce the rash slightly for short periods of time, but it recurs. On examination, there is an erythematous, macerated, eroded plaque in the inguinal folds extending to the scrotum and the medial thigh with surrounding scattered satellite papules and pustules (68).

68

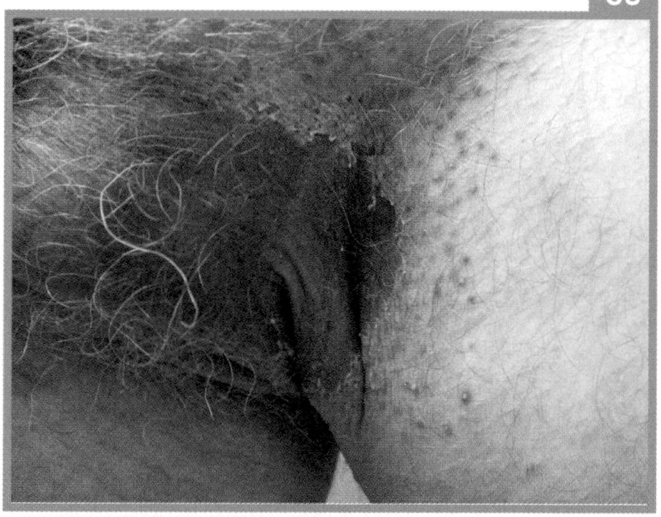

i. Which pathogen is responsible for this eruption?

ii. What other cutaneous manifestations can this pathogen produce?

iii. What populations are at higher risk of infection?

iv. What is the next best step in treatment?

Answer 68

i. Intertrigo is a commonly used term to define inflammation within the skin folds. Superimposed infection with *Candida* can occur in areas of occlusion and particularly after periods of prolonged immobilization. The most common candida species that cause mucocutaneous candidiasis are *Candida albicans* and *C. tropicalis.*

Candidal intertrigo usually involves the inguinal folds, between the buttocks, and/or inframammary folds. It classically presents with brightly erythematous irritable skin in moist areas that develops cracks or fissures. The rash is often sore and satellite papules, pustules or vesicles are often seen at the periphery. Candidiasis in the web spaces between the fingers is also known as erosio interdigitalis blastomycetica. It most commonly occurs between the third and fourth digits and is seen in individuals whose hands or feet are frequently exposed to water.

ii. In addition to intertrigo, candidal infections can produce a wide range of mucocutaneous manifestations, including oral candidiasis or oral thrush, angular cheilitis, vulvovaginal candidiasis in women, balanitis in men, chronic paronychia, onychomycosis and chronic mucocutaneous candidiasis (CMC).

CMC describes a group of disorders involving progressive and recurrent candidal infections of the skin, nails and mucous membranes with *C. albicans.* It is typically seen in patients with significant underlying immunologic abnormalities or autoimmune endocrinopathies.

iii. There are various predisposing factors for mucocutaneous candidiasis, including diabetes mellitus, occlusion or immobilization, hyperhidrosis, use of corticosteroids or antibiotics and immunosuppressed status.

CMC is observed in association with immunodeficiency disorders such as severe combined immunodeficiency, DiGeorge syndrome and hyper-IgE syndrome, as well as other non-immunologic inherited disorders such as keratitis ichthyosis deafness (KID) syndrome, multiple carboxylase deficiency, acrodermatitis enteropathica and ectodermal dysplasia–ectrodactyly–clefting syndrome. A subgroup of CMC occurs in the setting of autoimmune polyendocrinopathy–candidiasis–ectodermal dystrophy syndrome (APECED) and dectin-1 deficiency.

iv. The treatment of mucocutaneous candidal infections depends on the type of infection. Oral medications include fluconazole, itraconazole and nystatin (swish and swallow for oropharyngeal candidiasis). Topical treatments include clotrimazole, miconazole, tioconazole and nystatin. For candidal intertrigo or balanitis, topical imidazoles or ciclopirox can be used, with systemic agents reserved for recalcitrant or severe cases.

CMC does not typically respond to standard topical medications. Treatment usually requires long-term therapy with oral systemic antifungal agents.

CASE 69

Tinea corporis

QUESTION 69

A 37-year-old farmer presents with a pruritic rash affecting his buttocks and gluteal fold. He states that it has been present for approximately 7 days and has not responded to over-the-counter hydrocortisone cream. He initially presented with a single plaque that grew in size with central clearing, and then developed numerous other similar-appearing plaques nearby. On examination, there are annular and polycyclic plaques with an active erythematous and scaly border on the bilateral buttocks (69a).

69a

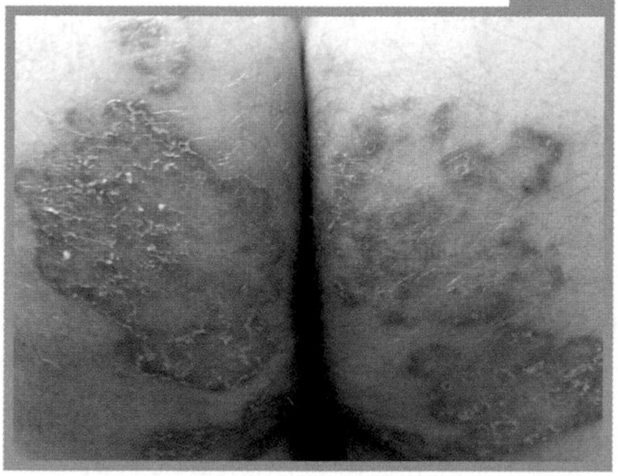

i. What is the most likely diagnosis?

ii. How can this diagnosis be distinguished from other diseases with similar presentation?

iii. What is the treatment?

Answer 69

i. The patient's rash is most consistent with tinea corporis, a superficial cutaneous fungal infection. Also known as dermatophytoses, these infections are caused by three genera of fungi (*Microsporum, Trichophyton, Epidermophyton*) that have the ability to infect keratinized tissue such as the hair, skin and nails. Named based on the anatomic area of involvement, tinea corporis refers to a dermatophyte infection of the trunk and extremities, excluding the hair, nails, acral surfaces and groin. Other dermatophyte infections include tinea pedis (soles and interdigital spaces), tinea manuum (palms and interdigital spaces), tinea cruris (inguinal region), tinea capitis (scalp), tinea barbae (bearded areas of the face and neck of men) and tinea unguium or onychomycosis (nails).

Tinea corporis can occur via human-to-human, animal-to-human or soil-to-human spread. Occupational or recreational exposures such as military housing, locker rooms, gymnasiums and outdoor occupations, as well as immunosuppressed states can predispose individuals to developing tinea corporis.

ii. Tinea corporis can often be mistaken for other eczematous conditions such as nummular eczema, atopic dermatitis and psoriasis, among others. Clinically, classic lesions of tinea corporis demonstrate an 'active' inflammatory border with scale, evidence of central clearing as the lesion progresses and failure to improve with topical steroids. Tinea incognito refers to cutaneous dermatophyte infections, which when treated with topical steroids can significantly reduce or eliminate scale, making the lesion more difficult to diagnose clinically. The diagnosis can be confirmed by potassium hydroxide (KOH) examination of a skin scraping demonstrating hyphae within the stratum corneum (69b) or histologically if a biopsy is obtained (positive periodic acid–Schiff [PAS] staining).

69b

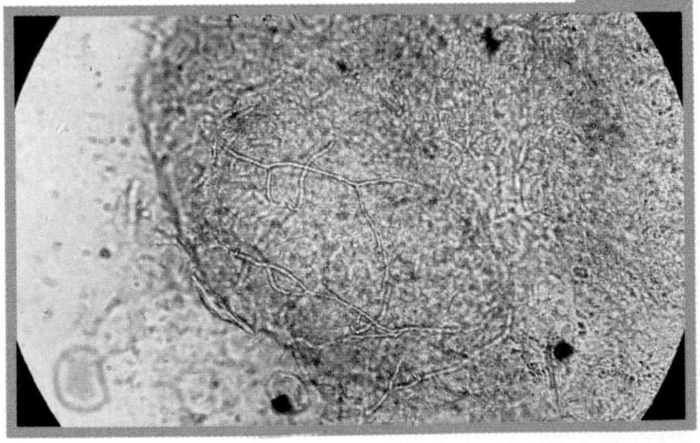

iii. The first-line treatment for uncomplicated, localized dermatophytoses is topical antifungals. Systemic antifungals such as fluconazole, griseofulvin, itraconazole or terbinafine can be used for dermatophyte infections involving extensive areas of the skin or associated with excessive inflammatory reactions.

CASE 70

Pityriasis versicolor

QUESTION 70

A 28-year-old man presents to the dermatology clinic with spreading red-brown spots on the face and trunk. The patient describes the dyspigmentation as slightly itchy, scaly and episodic, with flares in the warmer months and improvement over the winter. He was prescribed triamcinolone 0.1% ointment by his primary care provider but feels that this has made it worse. On examination, there are multiple light pink and light brown papules coalescing into plaques with subtle overlying scale (70a). Examination under a Wood's lamp reveals yellow-green fluorescence of the affected areas. Potassium hydroxide (KOH) preparation of a skin scraping reveals a 'spaghetti and meatball' presentation of spores and hyphal elements (70b). Fungal culture was negative.

70a

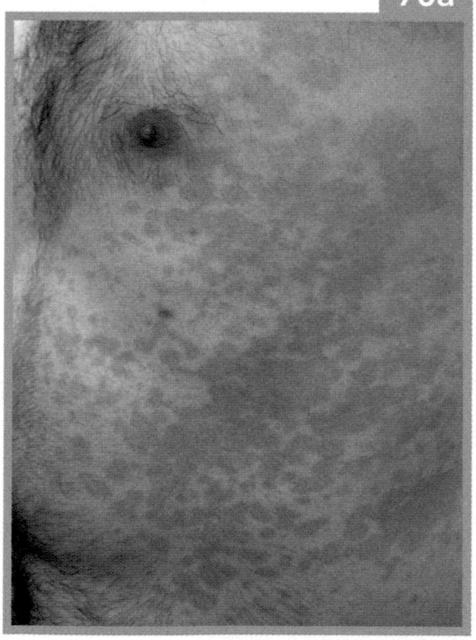

70b

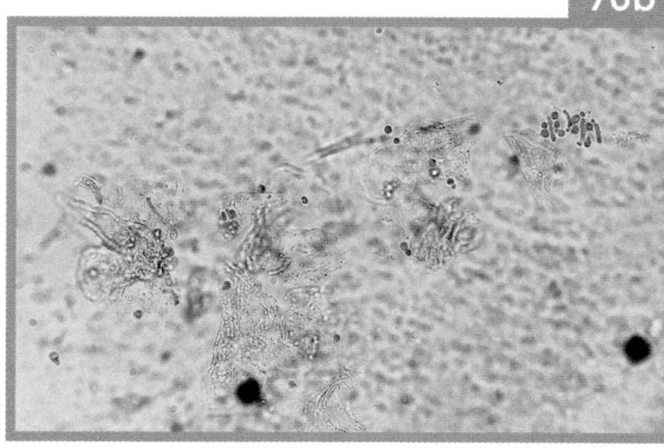

i. What is the diagnosis?

ii. What is the most likely causative organism?

iii. What are some of the risk factors?

Answer 70

i. This patient most likely has pityriasis versicolor, which usually presents with multiple round or oval thin plaques with overlying fine scales. The lesions can range from hypopigmented white-tan to hyperpigmented light brown or slightly erythematous pink plaques. They are distributed commonly over seborrheic areas, particularly the upper trunk and shoulders, and less often on the face, scalp, inframammary region and groin. Wood's lamp can be helpful to identify individual lesions, with yellow-green fluorescence seen in the affected areas. On KOH scraping, the classic findings are yeast and short mycelial forms, which have been referred to as 'spaghetti and meatballs' due to the appearance.

ii. The most likely causative organism is *Malassezia furfur.* The hypomelanosis which can be seen with pityriasis versicolor is thought to be due to the production of azelaic acid by *M. furfur*, which may contribute to decreased melanin synthesis.

iii. Risk factors for pityriasis versicolor include younger age, sweating, immunosuppression, oily skin and hot weather.

CASE 71

Blastomycosis

QUESTION 71

A 57-year-old woman presents to the dermatology clinic with an indolent painful ulcer on the abdomen. The patient reports associated symptoms of fever, chills, arthralgia, myalgia, night sweats and weight loss. On examination, there is a verrucous plaque with central ulceration and some granulation tissue on the abdomen (71a).

71a

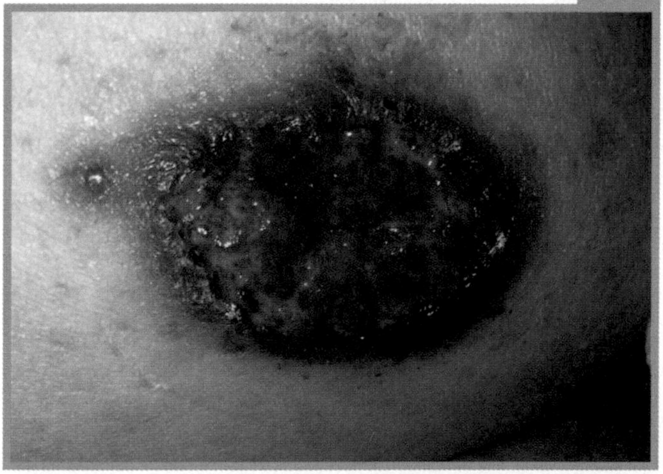

i. Does the cutaneous infection from this dimorphic fungus most commonly represent a primary infection or dissemination from a distant site?

ii. What is the most common primary site of infection?

iii. What is the treatment of choice?

iv. Which patient population is at higher risk for central nervous system (CNS) involvement, and what is the treatment of choice in this setting?

Answer 71

i. The patient presents with blastomycosis, a cutaneous infection caused by disseminated infection with the dimorphic fungus, *Blastomyces dermatitidis*. This disease is seen in the Mississippi and Ohio River valleys, Great Lakes and southeastern states of the United States. In its systemic form, it is seen most often in adult men, particularly those in occupations with outdoor exposure and/or frequent exposure to soil.

The cutaneous findings of blastomycosis are well-defined verrucous plaques with papules and pustules at the border, with central ulceration observed in advanced disease, which can resemble pyoderma gangrenosum.

ii. The most common primary site of infection is the lung (up to 70%), which occurs through inhalation of the causative organisms (71b). However, pulmonary infection can be subclinical in up to 50% of patients and cutaneous manifestations can be seen in the absence of pulmonary disease. Primary cutaneous infection is uncommon, occurring through direct inoculation of the skin through trauma.

71b

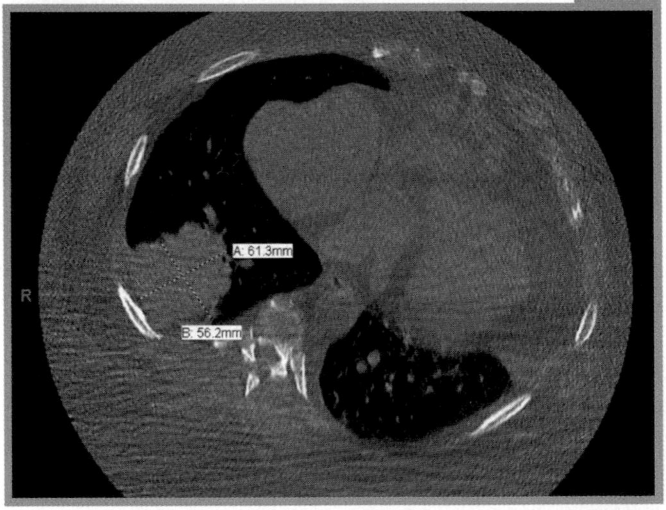

iii. The treatment of choice of blastomycosis is itraconazole. Alternative medications are ketoconazole and fluconazole.

iv. Immunocompromised patients have an increased risk of CNS involvement of blastomycosis (up to 40%). If disseminated disease involves the CNS, the treatment of choice is amphotericin B.

CASE 72

Aspergillosis

QUESTION 72

A 78-year-old man with a history of acute myeloid leukemia (AML) currently on induction chemotherapy was admitted to the hospital for the evaluation of fever and chills. He was neutropenic at the time of admission (with white blood cells [WBC] less than 0.5×10^9/L). Despite prompt initiation of broad-spectrum antibiotics, he became progressively hemodynamically unstable with hypotension and tachycardia and was subsequently intubated for acute hypoxic respiratory failure. Laboratory work-up demonstrated elevated lactic acid and serum inflammatory markers, but blood cultures drawn daily were all negative. On the third day of his hospital stay, the intensive care team consulted dermatology for evaluation of a necrotic lesion on the neck. On examination, there was a necrotic plaque on the right neck with surrounding erythema (72a). A skin biopsy was performed, which demonstrated septate hyphae with 45° angle branching and evidence of necrosis within blood vessels (72b).

72a

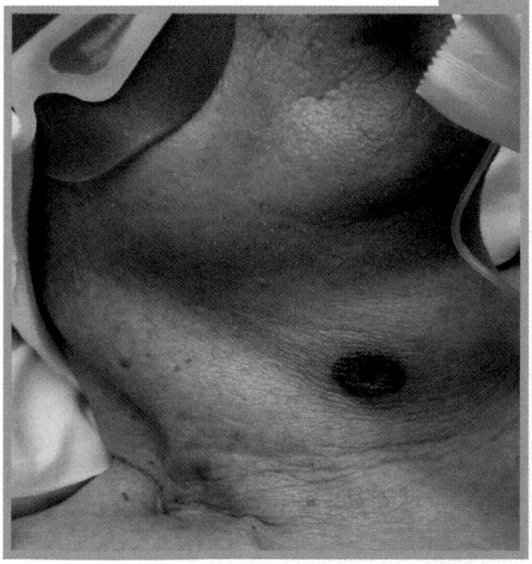

72b

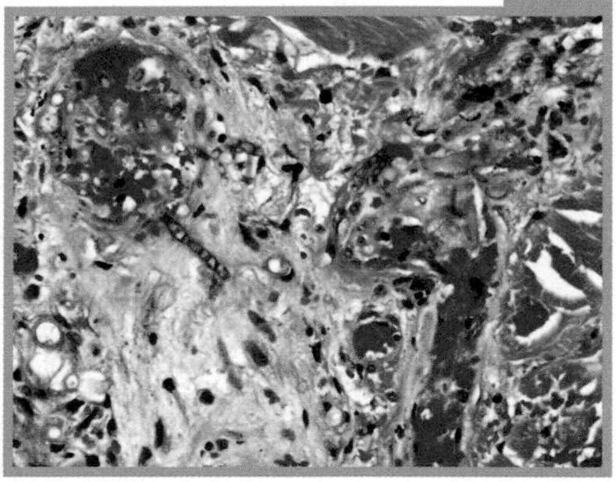

i. What is the diagnosis?

ii. What findings can be seen on histology to confirm the diagnosis?

iii. What is the treatment?

Answer 72

i. The patient presents with angioinvasive aspergillosis, which is an opportunistic fungal infection that is most often seen in immunocompromised populations, particularly in patients with advanced human immunodeficiency virus/acquired immunodeficiency syndrome (HIV/AIDS), AML, acute lymphoid leukemia and less often with myelodysplastic syndrome or other hematologic malignancies. The risk of developing angioinvasive aspergillosis is higher in patients undergoing hematopoietic stem cell transplantation or induction or consolidation chemotherapy. The most frequently identified pathogens are *Aspergillus fumigatus* and *A. flavus*, which can be difficult to identify in blood cultures but can be seen in histopathologic specimens. Clinically, aspergillosis is characterized by necrotic skin lesions that can be firm papules, papulonodules, hemorrhagic bullae or ulcers that develop due to the angioinvasive nature.

ii. On histology, narrow, non-pigmented, septate hyphae with 45° angle branching can be seen in the tissue. The fungi can invade the vessel walls causing tissue necrosis within the lumen.

iii. The prognosis is poor in disseminated aspergillosis, as internal organ involvement is often seen. Prophylactic treatment with systemic antifungals such as fluconazole or voriconazole can be administered to patients on myelosuppressive chemotherapy during periods of neutropenia. After the development of angioinvasive aspergillosis, treatment involves voriconazole, posaconazole or caspofungin.

DRUG-RELATED CUTANEOUS DISORDERS

CASE 73

Fixed drug reaction

QUESTION 73

A 47-year-old African American woman presents to the dermatology clinic for the evaluation of a recurrent rash on the right leg. She states that the rash began 3 months ago, shortly after she was treated with amoxicillin–clavulanate for a bacterial sinus infection. The rash seemed to improve after the infection resolved but since then, the rash has recurred at least once every 2–3 weeks. She believes that the rash returns in almost the exact spots on the body and does not seem to spread. On examination, there are two distinct, well-defined round violaceous plaques with a border of erythema on the right upper leg (73). She is otherwise healthy but does report occasional ibuprofen use for minor joint pain.

73

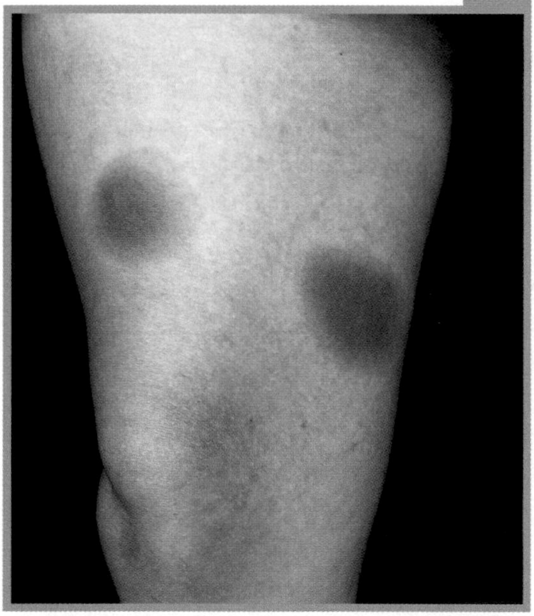

i. What is the diagnosis? What is the most likely cause of the patient's recurrent lesions?

ii. What should be considered on the differential diagnosis?

iii. What are the characteristic histopathologic findings of this condition?

Answer 73

i. The patient presents with a fixed drug eruption (FDE), which occurs approximately 1–2 weeks after exposure to a drug and is most frequently associated with sulfonamides, non-steroidal anti-inflammatory drugs (NSAIDs), barbiturates, tetracyclines and carbamazepine. It is characterized by the development of round, sharply demarcated erythematous and edematous plaques, sometimes with a violaceous centre or central bulla. They can occur anywhere on the body but favour the face, extremities and genitalia. A hallmark of FDE is the recurrence of lesions in the exact sites with readministration of the causative drug, with or without the development of additional sites of involvement. The most likely causative drug for this patient is the NSAID that she was taking, most likely for discomfort related to the sinusitis and then for joint pains thereafter.

ii. When there are multiple lesions of FDE, other entities to consider are erythema multiforme or Stevens–Johnson syndrome, particularly when there is oral mucosal involvement.

iii. On histopathological examination, biopsy specimens of FDE will demonstrate an interstitial and perivascular infiltrate consisting of lymphocytes, eosinophils and occasional neutrophils throughout the superficial and deep dermis. Dyskeratotic keratinocytes can be seen in the epidermis.

CASE 74

Acute generalized exanthematous pustulosis

QUESTION 74

A 57-year-old woman with a history of obesity, hypertension and type II diabetes mellitus is hospitalized with sepsis secondary to osteomyelitis. During her hospitalization, she develops fever and a diffuse erythematous rash with pustules that began on the face and axillae and then progressed to her trunk. Initial areas of involvement underwent superficial desquamation (74).

74

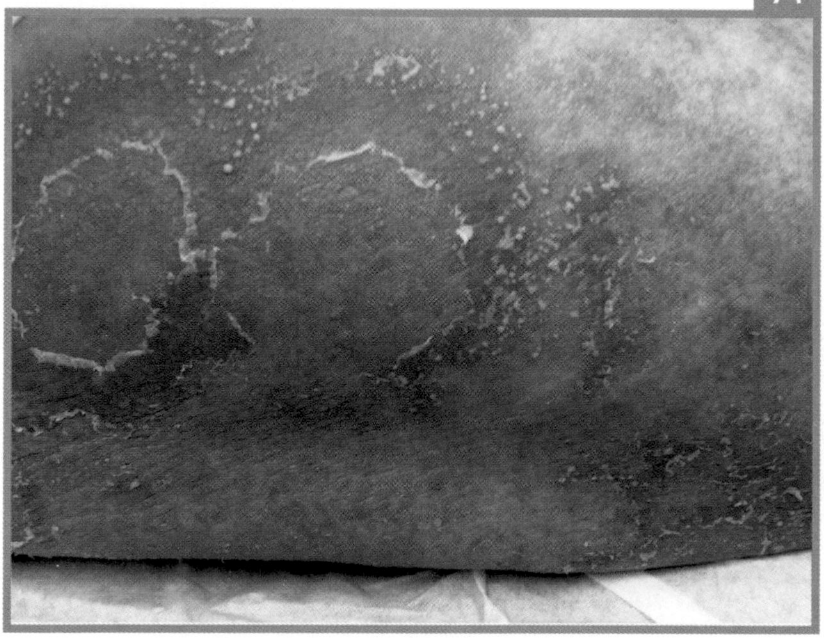

i. What is the diagnosis and aetiology?

ii. What is the other life-threatening rash that should be included on the differential diagnosis?

iii. What is the treatment for this condition?

Answer 74

i. Based on the history, morphologic features of the eruption and recent exposure to intravenous antibiotics for the treatment of osteomyelitis, the patient has developed acute generalized exanthematous pustulosis (AGEP), a febrile neutrophilic drug rash. AGEP is characterized by non-follicular, small, sterile pustules that tend to arise on the neck or flexural surfaces, which can disseminate over a course of hours. After 1–2 weeks, superficial desquamation is observed in the areas of involvement. Edema is seen in half of the patients, involving the face and hands. Vesicles, bullae and mucous membrane involvement are also commonly observed. Greater than 90% of the cases of AGEP are due to drugs, with the most common culprits being beta-lactam antibiotics and macrolides, followed by calcium channel blockers and antimalarials. Although the underlying mechanism of AGEP is still unknown, there are certain human leukocyte antigen (HLA) types that have been found at higher rates in patients with AGEP, including HLA-B5, HLA-DR11 and HLA-DQ3.

ii. The primary lesions of AGEP can be identical to the pustules seen in the von Zumbusch type of acute pustular psoriasis. In the latter entity, immediate medical care is imperative as this form of pustular psoriasis can be life-threatening, requiring intravenous fluids, topical and systemic treatment, including antibiotics. Patients with psoriasis tend to have a higher risk of developing AGEP, which can make the distinction even more challenging. Histologically, the presence of edema in the superficial dermis, exocytosis of eosinophils and necrosis of keratinocytes are suggestive of AGEP, in contrast to the acanthosis seen in pustular psoriasis.

iii. The treatment of AGEP involves withdrawal of the culprit medication(s), along with topical corticosteroids.

CASE 75

Stevens–Johnson syndrome/toxic epidermal necrolysis

QUESTION 75

A 71-year-old woman presents to the emergency room with fever, malaise and a peeling rash. She has a history notable for poorly controlled diabetes mellitus and had started a course of sulfamethoxazole–trimethoprim and ciprofloxacin for cellulitis of the right foot 8 days ago. On examination, there are large confluent areas of dusky erythema, flaccid bullae and denudation. There are also oral mucosal erosions around and inside the mouth and bilateral conjunctival injection. She is admitted to the hospital and continues to develop large confluent areas of dusky erythema on the trunk and extremities with a cigarette paper-like texture (75a) with new blister formation and progression of denudation (75b, c) involving 70% of the total body surface area.

75a

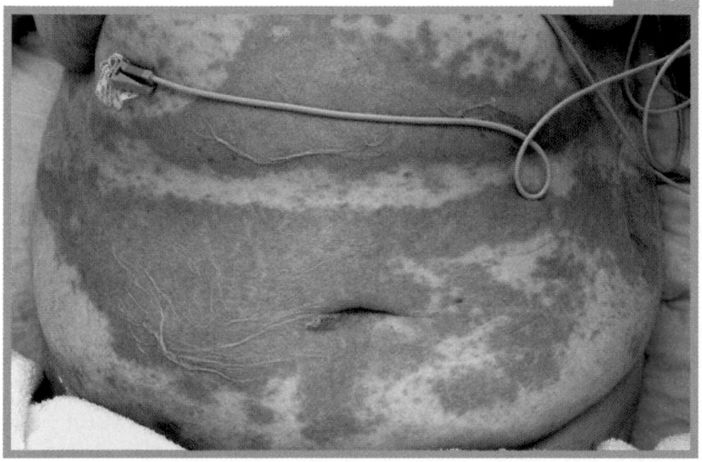

75b

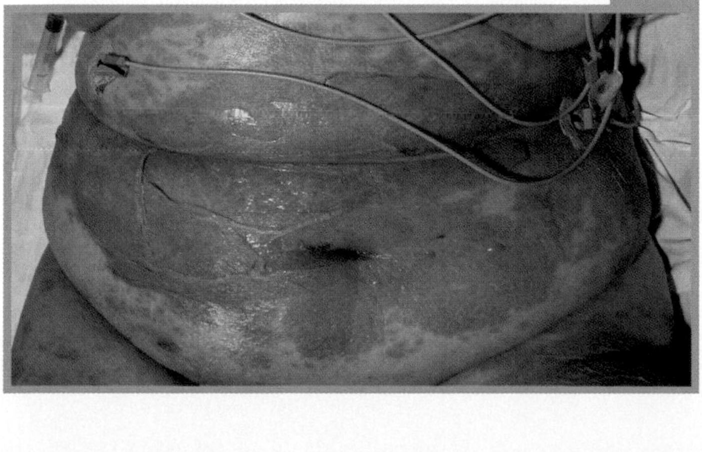

75c

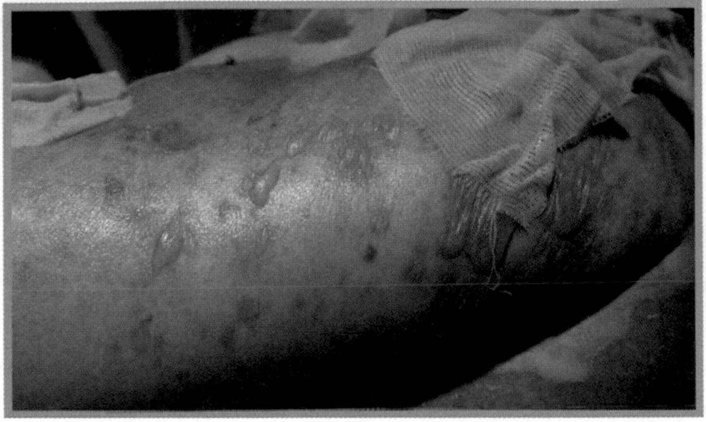

i. What is the diagnosis?

ii. What are the most common causes of this disorder, and what populations, if any, may be at risk?

iii. What are the complications and sequelae of this disease?

iv. What criteria can be used to predict mortality and what treatments are available?

Answer 75

i. The patient presents with toxic epidermal necrolysis (TEN), a severe mucocutaneous disease in the same spectrum as Stevens–Johnson syndrome (SJS). TEN has an average mortality between 25% and 35%. SJS/TEN is almost always due to drug exposures and is caused by massive keratinocyte death, which leads to separation of the skin at the dermal–epidermal junction. It presents typically with a prodrome of symptoms including fever, malaise, lymphadenopathy, pharyngitis and/or conjunctivitis, which can precede the skin findings by several days. The cutaneous manifestations of SJS/TEN include erythema and erosions that favour the trunk and face and later may involve the extremities. The oral, ocular and genital mucosae are involved in the vast majority of cases.

During progression of the disease, the erythematous patches appear dusky and may take on a grey hue that represents epidermal necrosis. Large areas of skin can resemble wet cigarette paper that sloughs off with minor friction or trauma (Nikolsky's sign). Flaccid blisters demonstrate the Asboe-Hansen sign, which is the extension of the blister sideways by slight pressure of the thumb due to the lateral displacement of necrotic epidermis.

The distinction between SJS and TEN is made upon the total body surface area (BSA) involved. SJS involves <10% of BSA, SJS/TEN overlap involves 10%–30% of BSA and TEN involves >30% of BSA.

ii. Medications that are most often associated with SJS/TEN include antimicrobials (aminopenicillins and trimethoprim–sulfamethoxazole), antiretroviral medications (particularly non-nucleoside reverse transcriptase inhibitors), allopurinol and anti-epileptic drugs (carbamazepine, phenytoin, lamotrigine and barbiturates).

SJS/TEN is a rare disease that has a slightly higher incidence in women. Populations at risk for developing SJS/TEN are those with slow acetylator genotypes, immunocompromised individuals or those undergoing radiotherapy, and patients on anticonvulsants. The risk of TEN is up to 1000-fold higher in individuals with AIDS than in the general population. In addition, specific human leukocyte antigen (HLA) alleles have been identified as higher risk. HLA-B*1502 in Asians and East Indians has been linked with a higher risk of SJS/TEN after exposure to carbamazepine, and HLA-B*5801 in Han Chinese has been linked with a higher risk after exposure to allopurinol.

iii. Areas of detached epidermis typically heal with re-epithelialization occurring within 3 weeks without any need for skin grafting. However, it is important to consult ophthalmology, gynecology and/or urology for the evaluation of mucosal involvement, as the manifestations on the mucosal surfaces can lead to sequelae such as symblepharon, conjunctival synechiae, entropion or blindness in the eyes and phimosis or vaginal synechiae in the genital mucosae.

iv. The SCORTEN scale is a severity-of-illness score that can be used in patients with TEN to predict mortality. It is based on seven independent risk factors for high mortality and is assessed at the time of presentation. One point is calculated for the presence of each of the seven parameters of the SCORTEN scale, which include age (>40 years), the presence of an associated malignancy, heart rate (>120 beats/min), total body surface area of epidermal detachment (>10% on day 1), serum urea level (>27 mg/dL), serum bicarbonate (<20 mEq/L) and serum glucose (>250 mg/dL).

SCORTEN	Mortality rate (%)
0–1	3.2
2	12.1
3	35.8
4	58.3
5+	90

Treatment of SJS/TEN includes the prompt removal of any or all potential offending drugs, admission to an intensive care unit (ICU) or burn unit with skilled nursing care, monitoring for fluid and electrolyte imbalances, maintenance of caloric intake and nutrition, and appropriate dressings to the denuded areas. There are no specific systemic treatments for SJS/TEN that have demonstrated efficacy in clinical trials, but several treatments have been reported in small case series, which include systemic corticosteroids, intravenous immunoglobulins (IVIg), cyclosporine, cyclophosphamide, plasmapheresis and anti-tumor necrosis factor-alpha (TNF-α) agents such as etanercept and infliximab.

CASE 76

Linear IgA bullous dermatosis

QUESTION 76

A 74-year-old woman with a history of chronic obstructive pulmonary disease presents to the hospital with fever, cough and shortness of breath. A chest X-ray demonstrates multifocal pneumonia and she is started on broad-spectrum antibiotics including vancomycin and piperacillin–tazobactam. During her hospitalization, she develops a bullous eruption on the trunk and dermatology is consulted. On examination, there are many tense vesicles and bullae on an erythematous base filled with serous fluid, some arranged in an arcuate pattern (76a).

76a

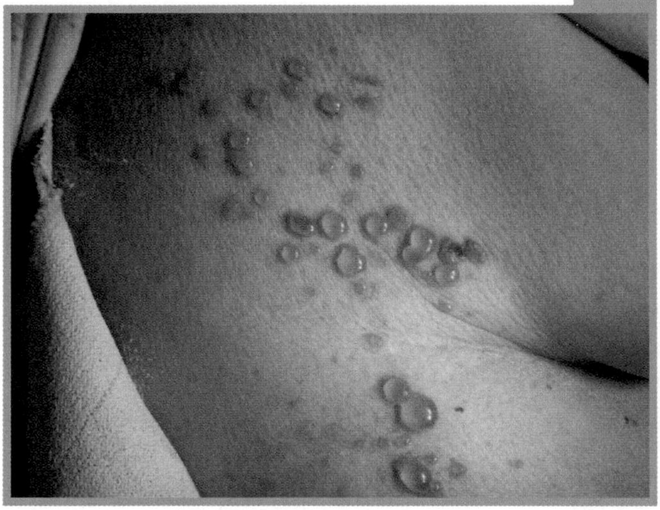

i. Based on this patient's history and clinical presentation, what is the diagnosis and what test should be used to confirm your suspicion?

ii. What is the treatment for this condition?

Answer 76

i. The patient has linear IgA bullous dermatosis (LABD), an immune-mediated bullous disorder characterized by subepidermal blisters and linear deposition of IgA along the basement membrane zone seen on direct immunofluorescence (76b). To confirm the diagnosis, a skin biopsy should be completed and sent for hematoxylin and eosin (H&E) stain as well as direct immunofluorescence. In adults, LABD is commonly drug induced. One of the most common culprit medications is vancomycin. Other drugs that have been identified in association with LABD are penicillins, cephalosporins, captopril and non-steroidal anti-inflammatory drugs (NSAIDs). LABD can also be idiopathic or seen in association with other disease processes including gastrointestinal disorders such as gluten-sensitive enteropathy and ulcerative colitis, infections and malignancies. There is a childhood form, known as chronic bullous disease of childhood, which is identical histologically to LABD but has a unique clinical presentation and has been associated with Crohn's disease but not medications or malignancy.

76b

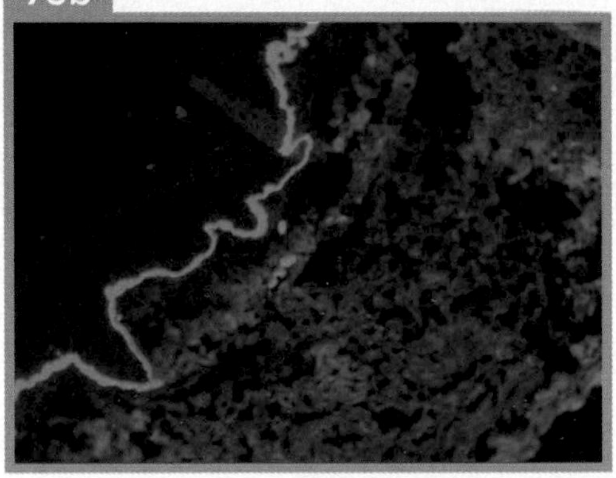

Clinically, LABD presents as subepidermal bullae arranged in a herpetiform or annular pattern. There are often clusters of smaller vesicles that are described as a 'crown of jewels' and new blisters tend to arise in a ring around older lesions, known as the 'string of beads' sign. In adults, the bullae often first present on the extremities and over time can progress to other sites. In children, the bullae classically involve the genital region initially but can spread to involve the face, lower trunk, hands and feet. Mucous membrane involvement is observed in up to 50% of patients.

ii. In patients with drug-induced LABD, the first step is to remove the offending agent. Most patients with LABD will respond further to oral dapsone therapy within 2–3 days. It is important to check the glucose-6-phosphate dehydrogenase (G-6-PD) level and adjust the dose accordingly. Sulfapyridine has also been used in place of dapsone. Oral prednisone up to 40 mg daily can also be used as an adjunctive treatment for disease control. Children usually respond to dapsone at a dose of 1–2 mg/kg daily.

CASE 77

Chemotherapy effects

QUESTION 77

A 79-year-old male with a history of metastatic melanoma in the lung and bone was found to have the V600K mutation and was started on treatment with a selective B-Raf murine sarcoma viral oncogene homolog B1 (BRAF) inhibitor, vemurafenib. Within a month after initiation of treatment, he presents to the dermatology clinic for the evaluation of tense bullae on the lateral aspects of the hands, painful hyperkeratotic papules of the face and ears, along with a seborrheic dermatitis-like eruption on the face (77a–c).

77a

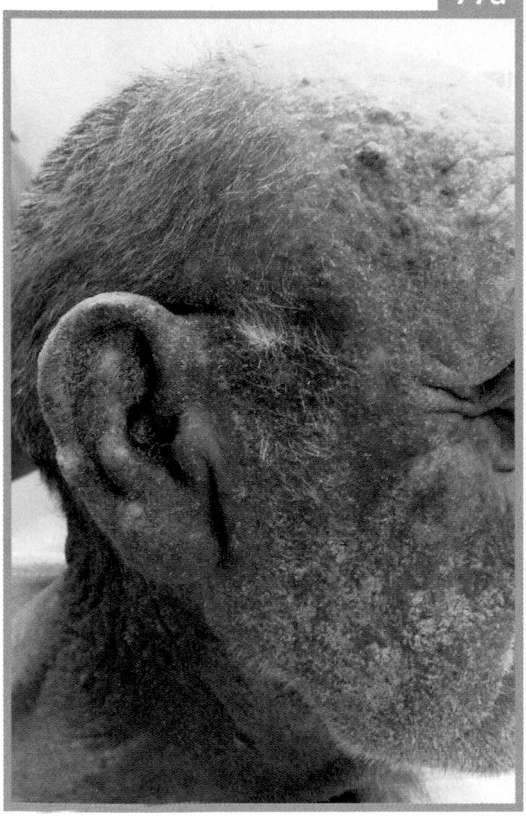

77b

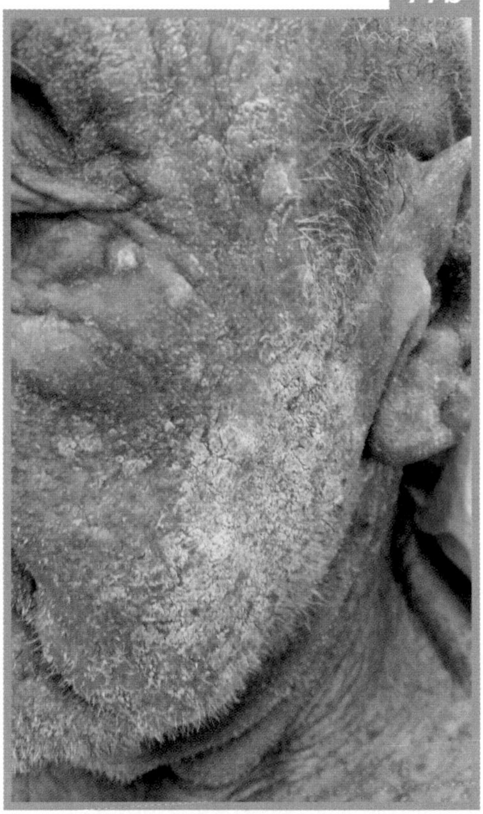

77c

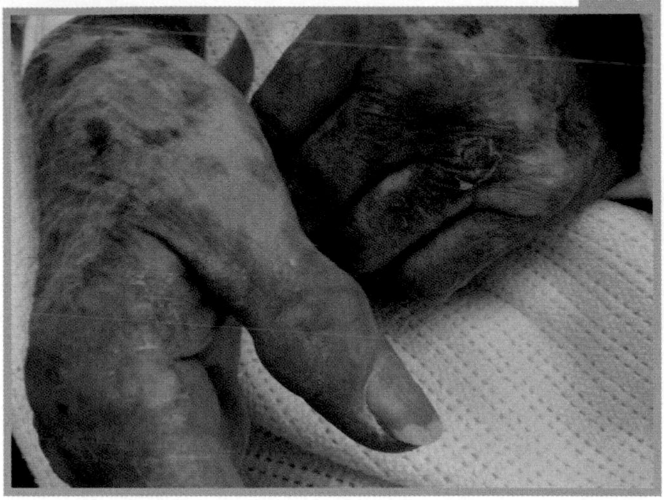

i. What is the cause of this patient's cutaneous eruption?

ii. What are the potential treatments?

Answer 77

i. This patient presents with a cutaneous adverse reaction to vemurafenib, a BRAF inhibitor. Cutaneous side effects can be seen in up to 58% of patients treated with vemurafenib, with up to 42% of patients having more than one skin-related complication. The most common cutaneous side effects of vemurafenib include hyperkeratotic eruptions, verrucous papillomas, facial erythema, seborrheic dermatitis, cystic lesions, phototoxic reactions after ultraviolet (UV) exposure, alopecia and hand-foot skin reactions. Patients may also present with eruptive squamous cell carcinomas and actinic keratoses. This patient is presenting with multiple cutaneous side effects after initiation of vemurafenib. On the face, there is an eruption of verrucous and hyperkeratotic lesions on UV-exposed skin, including the face and ears, as well as the eruption of actinic keratoses and squamous cell carcinomas. The patient also has hand-foot syndrome, characterized by erythema, edema and desquamation of the palms and soles.

ii. For individual lesions, cryotherapy or excision of unresponsive or painful lesions can be performed. Topical treatment with steroids such as mometasone furoate has been used to treat the general eruption, with clearing seen within 2–4 weeks. The use of urea-based ointments for hydration can help prevent the relapse of lesions. In a patient with eruptive squamous cell carcinomas and actinic keratoses, isotretinoin and 5-fluorouracil were used to clear these lesions. In hand-foot syndrome, discontinuation of the offending agent often leads to resolution of the symptoms.

CASE 78

Flagellate hyperpigmentation

QUESTION 78

A 41-year-old man presents to the dermatology clinic for the evaluation of dark linear lesions on his back. He has a medical history of chronic kidney disease (stage II), alcohol dependency and Hodgkin's lymphoma, for which he is currently undergoing treatment. He states that the rash developed over 3 days and was initially extremely pruritic. On examination, there are linear hyperpigmented streaks across the back with few scattered excoriations (78).

78

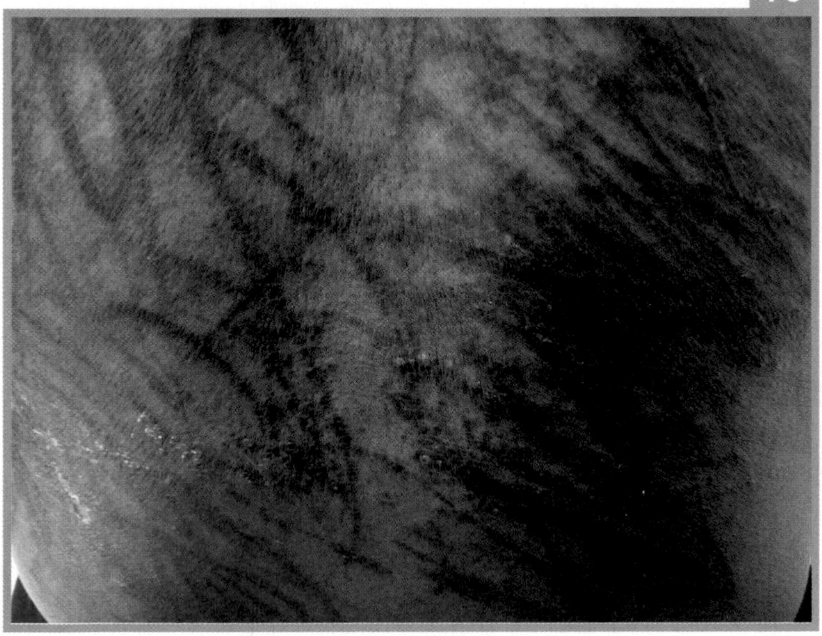

i. What is the most likely diagnosis?

ii. What are the other cutaneous findings can be seen that are associated with this condition?

iii. What are the other causes of similar cutaneous findings?

iv. What is the disease course and treatment?

Answer 78

i. The patient's clinical presentation and medical history of Hodgkin's lymphoma on chemotherapy is supportive of a diagnosis of flagellate pigmentation from bleomycin. Bleomycin is a cytotoxic antibiotic used to treat malignancies such as Hodgkin's lymphoma, non-Hodgkin's lymphoma, as well as testicular, ovarian and cervical cancers. In up to 20% of patients treated with systemic bleomycin, flagellate hyperpigmentation can occur, usually in a dose-dependent manner. The pigmentation can appear within 1 day to 9 weeks after drug administration, but typically after cumulative doses of 100–300 mg.

ii. Bleomycin is associated with additional cutaneous side effects, including painful nodules on the fingers, verrucous plaques on the knees and elbows and Raynaud's phenomenon. Nail changes can also be seen in patients treated with bleomycin, including melanonychia, Beau's lines, onychomadesis and onycholysis.

iii. Shiitake mushroom dermatitis can also present with similar flagellate lesions in the setting of ingestion or exposure to raw shiitake mushrooms. Flagellate erythema can also occur in patients with dermatomyositis and adult-onset Still's disease.

iv. There is no specific therapy for bleomycin-related flagellate hyperpigmentation. Symptom management with topical corticosteroids and oral antihistamines can be used. The pigmentation tends to fade over the course of months after bleomycin is discontinued.

CONGENITAL LESIONS AND LESIONS OF NEWBORNS

CASE 79

Erythema toxicum neonatorum

QUESTION 79

A 4-day-old full-term neonate is seen in the pediatric dermatology clinic for a spreading rash. The patient's mother states the skin changes started just after bringing him home from the hospital. His mother does note that the spots she initially observed on day 1 of the rash have subsequently resolved, but have been replaced by numerous new spots. The infant is otherwise healthy and the areas do not seem to be itchy or painful. On examination, there are numerous splotchy red macules with central yellow or white pustules (79).

79

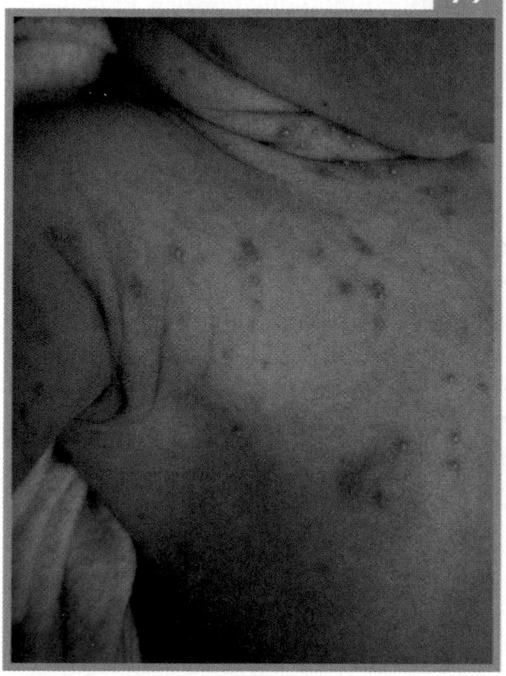

i. What is the most likely diagnosis?

ii. What other diseases should be considered on the differential diagnosis?

iii. What inflammatory cell is noted microscopically on scraping of a pustule?

iv. What are the characteristic features of this disease on histopathological examination?

v. What is the treatment of choice for this condition?

Answer 79

i. Based on this patient's presentation, the diagnosis is erythema toxicum neonatorum (ETN). A common vesiculopustular eruption in neonates, ETN is seen in up to 50% of full-term neonates and presents in most cases within 24–48 hours after delivery. Various combinations of erythematous macules, wheals, pustules, vesicles or papules can be seen in different stages of healing. Lesions may wax and wane over several days, and mechanical irritation can precipitate new lesions. ETN typically involves the face, trunk and limbs, while sparing the palms and soles.

ii. The differential diagnosis includes other pustular disorders of newborns, such as bacterial infections (staphylococcal and streptococcal infections), candidiasis, herpesvirus infections, scabies, transient neonatal pustular melanosis, miliaria, neonatal cephalic pustulosis, eosinophilic pustular folliculitis, congenital Langerhans cell histiocytosis, incontinentia pigmenti, hyper-IgE syndrome, and neonatal Behçet's disease.

iii. On scraping of a pustule, Wright's stain of the pustular contents will demonstrate numerous eosinophils, which can help confirm the diagnosis.

iv. On histologic examination, the outer root sheaths of hair follicles are infiltrated by eosinophils, with coalescing subcorneal pustules with eosinophils seen in a perifollicular distribution.

v. Erythema toxicum neonatorum is a benign eruption and individual lesions typically resolve within days. The rash is asymptomatic and heals without scarring, requiring no therapy.

CASE 80

Accessory tragus

QUESTION 80

An 8-year-old Asian girl presents to the clinic with her parents due to a concern about a skin-coloured, firm protrusion near her ear. It has been present since birth and does not cause any symptoms, but can be painful with minor trauma and putting on clothing. On examination, there is a firm, exophytic skin-coloured growth in the preauricular area with a firm stalk-like base (80).

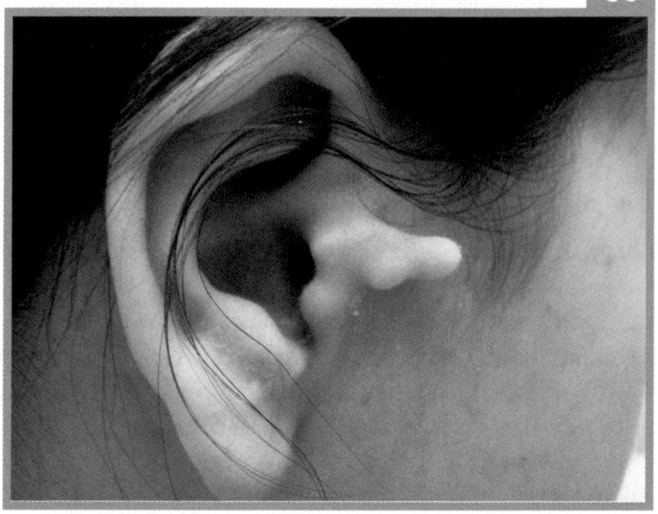

80

i. What is the diagnosis?

ii. What are the characteristic features on histology?

iii. What other condition does this overlap with?

iv. What syndrome(s) is this associated with?

Answer 80

i. This patient has an accessory tragus, also known as a preauricular tag. This is a relatively common benign congenital anomaly. It is a cartilaginous projection that is usually located anterior to the external auditory meatus. Accessory tragi are derived from the first branchial arch and may signal a defect in the first or second branchial arches. They should be distinguished from skin tags (acrochordon), and care should be taken when performing a biopsy, as removal may expose cartilage, causing slow healing or even chondrodermatitis nodularis chronica helicis.

ii. Histologically, an accessory tragus is polypoid, with a normal or thin stratum corneum, rugated epidermal surface with a central cartilaginous core. Vellus hair follicles, as well as adipose tissue and dilated blood vessels can be seen in the papillary dermis.

iii. An accessory tragus is thought to overlap with the hair follicle nevus (also known as vellus hamartoma), a congenital hamartoma of hairs and follicles, usually on the face and commonly near the ear. Some have suggested that these two entities are the same, as they exhibit identical patterns microscopically.

iv. Less commonly, accessory tragi can be a sign of other syndromes. Oculoauricularvertebral dysplasia (Goldenhar's syndrome) is one in which accessory tragi are a constant feature. Goldenhar's syndrome includes accessory tragi, epibulbar desmoids and vertebral defects. It is associated with the anomalous development of the first and second branchial arches. Accessory tragi can also be seen in Townes–Brocks, Treacher–Collins, VACTERL (vertebral anomalies, anal atresia, cardiac defects, tracheoesophageal fistula, esophageal atresia, renal and radial anomalies and limb defects) and Wolf–Hirschhorn syndrome.

CASE 81

Congenital nevus

QUESTION 81

A 13-week-old boy presents to the pediatric dermatology clinic for the evaluation of a dark lesion on his back, present since birth. His mother states that the lesion covered most of his back since birth, and has continued to grow in size proportionally with the child. On examination, there is a large brown-blue lesion covering much of the back, with areas of thickened papules and diffuse thin hairs throughout the lesion (81).

81

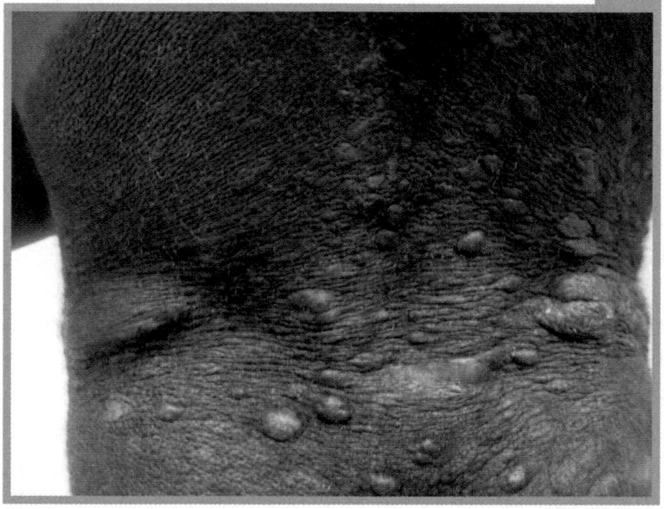

i. What is the diagnosis?

ii. What additional tests are recommended?

iii. What are the risks associated with this congenital lesion?

iv. What are the treatment options?

Answer 81

i. This patient presents with a giant congenital melanocytic nevus. Congenital nevi are categorized by the final size in adults defined as small nevi <1.5 cm in diameter, medium congenital nevi between 1.5 and 19.9 cm, and large or giant congenital nevi >20 cm in diameter. In newborns, nevi at least 9 cm on the scalp and 6 cm on the trunk are considered to be giant congenital nevi. Some have described a fourth category for nevi >40 cm in diameter in adults, also known as the garment nevi. These melanocytic nevi, as the name implies, are present at birth and consist of proliferations of benign melanocytes. The estimated incidence of giant congenital nevi is 0.005%. Over time, congenital melanocytic nevi can acquire a pebbled surface with raised areas, colour darkening and papules and nodules, also known as proliferative nodules.

ii. Neurocutaneous melanosis is observed at a higher frequency in patients with giant congenital melanocytic nevi, especially in nevi with a posterior axial location involving the head, neck, back and/or buttocks. Neurocutaneous melanosis can be either asymptomatic or symptomatic, with signs of increased intracranial pressure due to hydrocephalus or mass effect. On magnetic resonance imaging (MRI), neurocutaneous melanosis can present with multiple postgadolinium-enhancing masses, diffusely thickened leptomeninges or focal areas of increased signal on T1-weighted images.

iii. All congenital melanocytic nevi can be associated with melanoma, but the risk of melanoma is higher in larger melanocytic nevi. Across several large-scale studies, the risk of developing primary cutaneous melanoma within giant congenital nevi ranges from 2.5% to 12%. In patients with neurocutaneous melanosis, leptomeningeal melanomas can arise, usually involving the frontal and temporal lobes, and are associated with very poor prognosis.

iv. For small- and medium-sized melanocytic nevi, routine excision is typically not recommended due to the low melanoma risk associated with these lesions. However, some may seek treatment due to the cosmetic appearance or location of the nevus. For the treatment of giant congenital nevi, treatment can be more challenging. Excision is typically delayed until at least 6 months of age. Excision for large lesions on the back such as in this patient is usually performed in stages. Other potential treatment options include dermabrasion, repeat curettage or laser treatment. However, scarring, prolonged healing and recurrence of pigmentation are drawbacks to these methods.

CASE 82

Supernumerary nipple

QUESTION 82

A 51-year-old man presents to the dermatology office for a full-body skin check-up. He has no personal or family history of skin cancer. He is concerned about multiple growths on his arms and back. He also would like a brown colour growth on his right upper abdomen checked. It has been present since childhood but he noticed a new growth near to that area. On physical examination, there is a brown patch inferior to the right areola with an overlying small pink-brown papule (82).

82

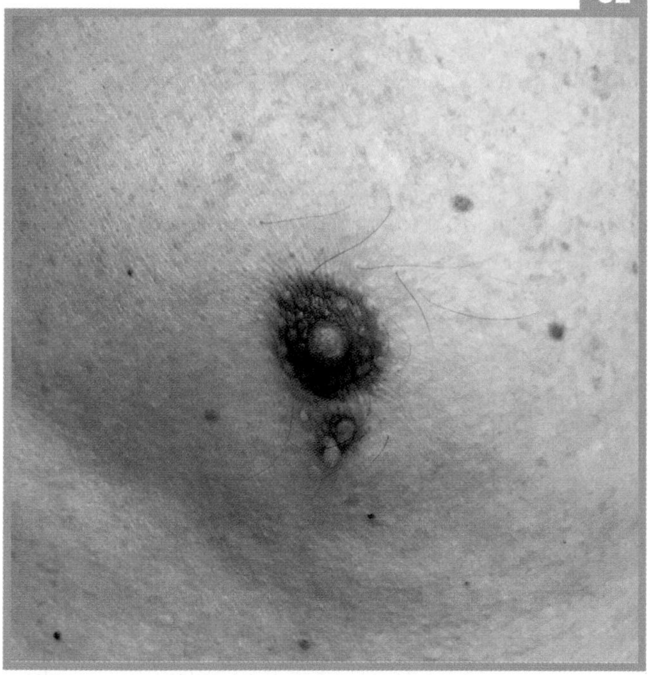

i. What is the diagnosis and what is this lesion embryologically derived from?

ii. What are some other lesions or conditions associated with this clinical finding?

iii. What are the histologic features of this lesion?

Answer 82

i. The lesion is a supernumerary nipple, also known as an accessory nipple. It is an embryological remnant of the mammary ridges or milk lines, which are derived from the ectoderm. They can be located anywhere along the milk lines, which run bilaterally along the axilla, breast, lateral abdomen and groin. Supernumerary nipples are usually a sporadic developmental anomaly, although up to 10% are familial.

As supernumerary nipples represent ectopic mammary tissue, they can demonstrate functional features similar to normal breasts, including tenderness and swelling during menstruation in women.

ii. In patients with supernumerary nipples, there is an increased incidence of Becker's nevi. Few studies have also found that supernumerary nipples occur at a higher incidence in patients with urogenital or renal cancers. There are also congenital syndromes in which supernumerary nipples are found, which include Simpson–Golabi–Behmel syndrome, ectodermal dysplasia cleft lip/palate syndrome and tricho-odonto-onychial dysplasia.

iii. Histologically, supernumerary nipples will demonstrate features similar to normal mammary tissue, including pilosebaceous structures, smooth muscle and mammary glands. They can also potentially develop disorders seen in normal mammary tissue, such as fibrocystic changes, fibroadenomas and carcinomas.

CASE 83

Nevus sebaceous

QUESTION 83

A 25-year-old man presents for the evaluation of a growth on his scalp. Although it has been present since birth, he is concerned about the appearance and reports that it is occasionally tender with minor trauma. On examination, there is a large plaque with a yellow-orange hue located on the scalp with a pebbly surface (83).

83

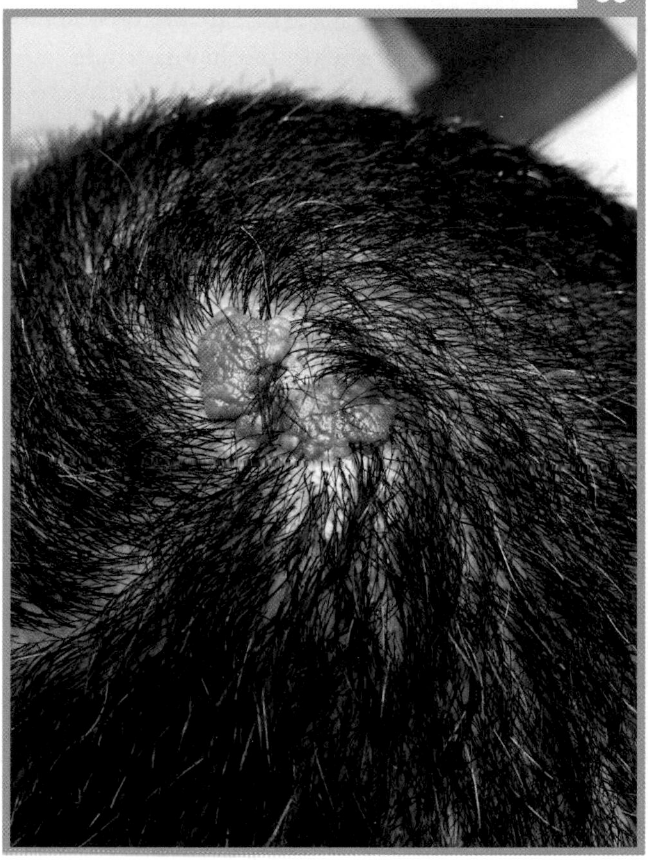

i. What is the most likely diagnosis of this case?

ii. What are the characteristic features of this lesion on histopathological examination?

iii. What additional concerns should be raised about this lesion?

Answer 83

i. This patient's lesion is a nevus sebaceous, a non-neoplastic malformation that includes follicular, sebaceous and apocrine elements. They appear at birth as small, slightly raised lesions, usually occurring on the scalp, face or neck. On the scalp, hair growth occurs around the lesion. Over time, the nevus sebaceous becomes thicker and pebbly with verrucous changes of the overlying skin being common.

ii. On histology, early childhood lesions will show small misshapen follicular lesions. In lesions of later adolescence and adulthood, there is epidermal acanthosis and fibroplasia of the papillary dermis, as well as enlarged sebaceous glands in the epidermal–dermal junction.

iii. Previously, it was thought that secondary carcinomas could occur within a nevus sebaceous. However, it is now thought that most secondary proliferations are benign follicular neoplasms, such as trichoblastomas and syringocystadenomas. The actual incidence of a secondary malignancy such as basal cell carcinomas is less than 1%.

CASE 84

Nevus comedonicus

QUESTION 84

A 4-year-old girl presents to the pediatric dermatology office as a referral for changes on the left forearm that have been present since birth. According to the patient's mother, the area appears to be spreading over the last year. There have been no treatments prior to this presentation. On physical examination, there are closely grouped slightly elevated papules with central black keratinous plugs as well as a few inflammatory papules in a linear unilateral distribution that follows the lines of Blaschko (84a, b).

84a

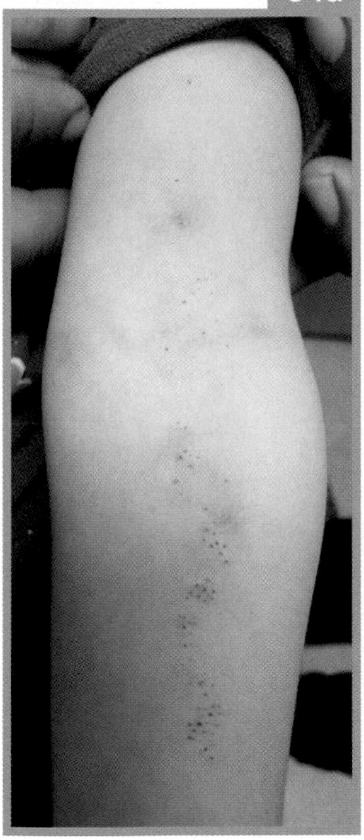

84b

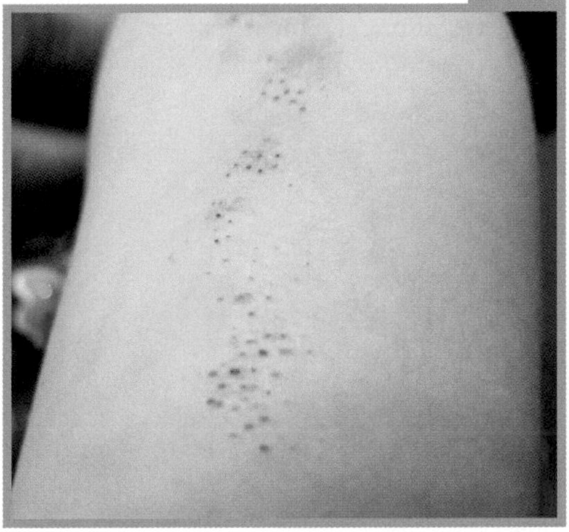

i. What is the gene mutation for this condition?

ii. What is the natural history of this condition?

Answer 84

i. Nevus comedonicus is an epidermal nevus that has been associated with a mutation in the fibroblast growth factor receptor 2 (*FGFR2*) gene. Nevus comedonicus is a genetic mosaicism; however, it is allelic (same gene mutation) to Apert syndrome, a somatic or autosomal dominantly inherited condition with craniosynostosis, syndactyly, midface hypoplasia and early-onset severe acne. Like other epidermal nevi, nevus comedonicus can be rarely associated with systemic findings, such as skeletal and central nervous system (CNS) anomalies.

ii. Nevus comedonicus is composed of a collection of dilated hair follicles filled with keratin. They are usually present at birth or develop during early childhood. There can be rapid growth at puberty with the development of inflammatory acne lesions. Medical treatment options include topical retinoids, salicylic acid and ammonium lactate. For severe or disfiguring nevi, ablative laser or surgical management may be considered.

CASE 85

Angiokeratoma circumscriptum

QUESTION 85

A 3-year-old girl presents to the pediatric dermatology office as a referral for the evaluation of an enlarging vascular growth on her leg. The patient's mother states that she initially thought it was a bruise but noticed that it slowly grew larger instead of regressing over time. It does not seem to bother the child. On physical examination, it was found that there is a plaque of grouped blue-purple papules on the left thigh that are confluent in some areas (85).

85

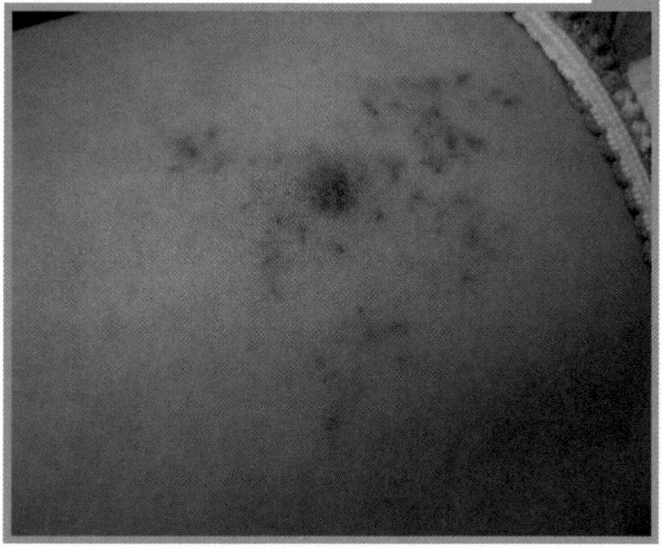

i. What are the five variants of this lesion? How does this lesion differ from other variants?

ii. What congenital disease(s) is/are associated with the development of multiple lesions?

iii. What are the treatment options?

Answer 85

i. Angiokeratomas are vascular lesions that result from the dilation of superficial vessels. They are usually well-circumscribed and can have variable levels of hyperkeratosis. There are five variants of angiokeratomas: solitary or multiple angiokeratomas, angiokeratomas of the scrotum or vulva (also known as angiokeratoma of Fordyce), angiokeratoma corporis diffusum, angiokeratoma of Mibelli and angiokeratoma circumscriptum. This patient presents with angiokeratoma circumscriptum, which typically develops in infancy or childhood and favours the trunk, arms or legs in a unilateral distribution. This variant differs from the other types of angiokeratomas because it can be the result of a lymphatic capillary or capillary malformation, whereas all other variants of angiokeratomas represent an ectatic dilation of pre-existing vessels in the papillary dermis.

Solitary or multiple angiokeratomas present as small, warty, black papules that favour the lower extremities but can occur anywhere on the body. Clinically, they can be confused with melanoma due to the dark colour. Angiokeratomas of Fordyce are characterized by multiple red, purple or black papules arising along superficial vessels on the vulva or scrotum. These are typically seen in older age groups, but can be observed as early as the second decade. Vulvar lesions are associated with oral contraceptive use and increased venous pressure during pregnancy. Angiokeratoma corporis diffusum is characterized by the development of multiple angiokeratomas on the body, often in a bathing suit distribution. Angiokeratomas of Mibelli usually occur on the dorsal and lateral aspects of the hands and feet, and are associated with chilblains and acrocyanosis.

ii. Angiokeratoma corporis diffusum usually develops during late childhood or adolescence and presents as clusters of angiokeratomas on the trunk and bathing suit distribution. It can be linked with multiple inherited metabolic disorders but is most commonly associated with Fabry disease, an X-linked recessive disease caused by a deficiency in the lysosomal enzyme α-galactosidase A. Other associated disorders include aspartylglycosaminuria (deficiency in aspartylglycosaminidase), GM1 gangliosidosis (deficiency in β-galactosidase), fucosidosis (deficiency in α-fucosidase) and sialidosis (deficiency in sialidase).

iii. Angiokeratomas are benign and do not require removal. However, if patients request removal for cosmetic purposes, surgical options include laser therapy, cryotherapy, electrocautery and excision, depending on the location and size of the lesions.

GENODERMATOSES

CASE 86

Aplasia cutis congenita

QUESTION 86

An 18-month-old boy presents to the dermatology clinic with his mother for the evaluation of an area without hair growth on the vertex of the scalp, which has been present since birth. The area is asymptomatic, but the patient's mother is concerned about the hair loss. On examination, there is a patch of scarring alopecia on the vertex of the scalp with a slightly atrophic centre (86).

86

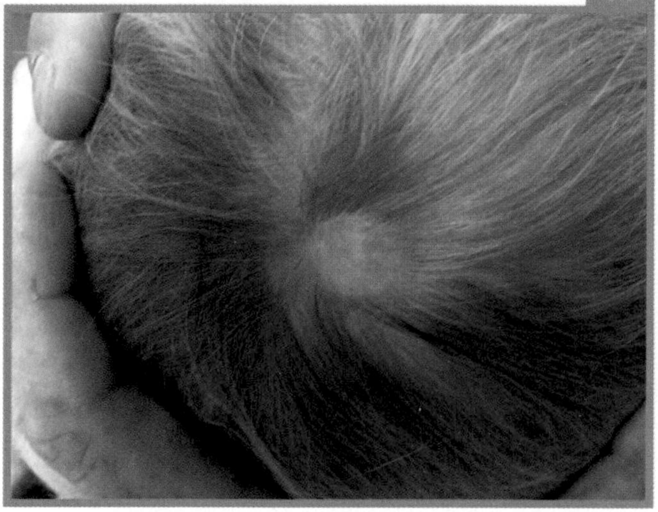

i. What is the diagnosis?

ii. What other syndromes can be seen with this lesion?

Answer 86

i. This patient has aplasia cutis congenita (ACC), also known as cutis aplasia or congenital scars. This is a skin condition present at birth characterized by absent or scarred areas of the skin. It is caused by abnormal intrauterine skin development, which may be the consequence of a variety of factors including genetic factors, vascular factors, trauma, teratogens or intrauterine infection. ACC is one of the skin lesions of the spinal axis associated with dysraphism. When seen in combination with other skin lesions of the spinal axis, such as an infantile hemangioma, connective tissue nevus, congenital melanocytic nevus or dimples, there is an increased risk of an underlying spinal anomaly and further work-up should be performed.

ACC can demonstrate a wide range of clinical presentations. The patient in this case presents with the most common form, known as membranous aplasia cutis. Membranous lesions typically occur on the midline scalp and present initially at birth as a sharply demarcated round defect with a surrounding collarette of hair, covered by a translucent shiny epithelial membrane. Over time, the lesion flattens to form an atrophic scar. Another major type of ACC is characterized by the presence of stellate lesions that often demonstrate ulceration with a raw hemorrhagic or granulating base.

The scalp accounts for >85% of lesions of ACC. Scalp ACC without other anomalies is usually present at the vertex near the parietal hair whorl. Patients can also present with multiple membranous lesions in a linear arrangement.

ii. There are several syndromes associated with scalp ACC. One notable syndrome is Adams–Oliver syndrome, which usually follows an autosomal dominant inheritance pattern. The associated ACC lesions can be large and irregular, and are usually located on the midline scalp along with skull defects and dilated scalp veins. In addition, terminal transverse limb defects, cutis marmorata telangiectatica congenita, cardiac malformations and central nervous system abnormalities are observed. ACC can also be seen in patients with Goltz syndrome and several types of ectodermal dysplasias.

CASE 87

Incontinentia pigmenti

QUESTION 87

A 3-month-old infant girl presents with her mother to the pediatric dermatology clinic for the evaluation of blisters on the arms and upper chest. Her mother states that the blisters have been present for about 3 days, and her pediatrician was concerned about scabies infestation and had treated her and all family members with permethrin 5% cream with no improvement. On examination, there is a linear arrangement of erythematous vesicles and bullae on the arms and upper chest (87). A single vesicle was unroofed and Tzanck smear was negative.

87

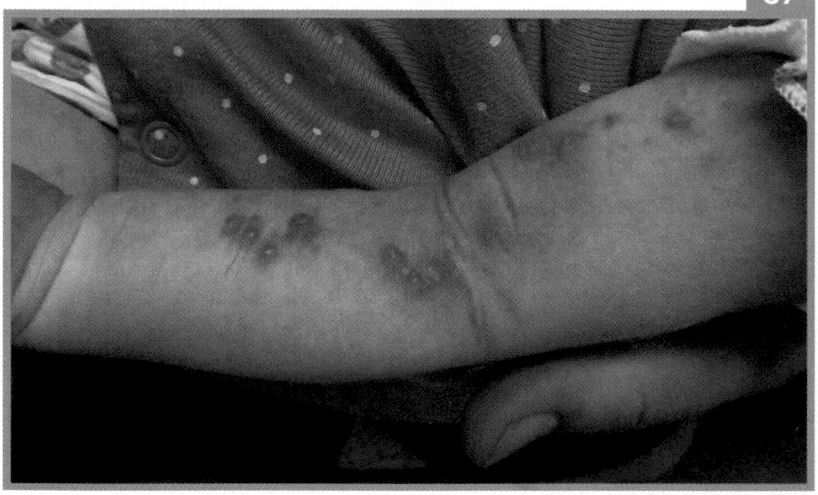

i. What is the most likely diagnosis?

ii. What is the gene defect and how can this disease occur in males?

iii. What other disorder(s) is this gene defect seen in?

iv. What is the clinical progression of these lesions?

v. What are the associated findings in this disorder?

vi. What other specialists should be involved in the management of this patient?

Answer 87

i. The most likely diagnosis is incontinentia pigmenti (IP), also known as Bloch–Sulzberger syndrome, which is a rare X-linked dominant multisystem disorder. Although it can appear similar to infectious aetiologies such as scabies infestation, herpes simplex or varicella infections, neonatal IP has a characteristic pattern of skin lesions that follow a linear Blaschko pattern. The linearity of the skin lesions is a result of mosaicism due to lionization or X-inactivation.

ii. IP is an X-linked dominant disorder caused by mutations in the *NEMO* gene located at Xq28. The NEMO protein plays a role in tumour necrosis factor-alpha (TNF-α)-induced apoptosis. Although it is typically lethal in males, clinical IP can occasionally be seen in boys with Klinefelter syndrome (XXY) or in boys with genomic mosaicism from a half-chromatid or post-zygotic mutation.

iii. Mutations in the *NEMO* gene are also seen in hypohidrotic ectodermal dysplasia with immune deficiency.

iv. There are four different recognized stages of lesions of IP: vesicular, verrucous, hyperpigmented and hypopigmented/atrophic. Initially, IP presents with vesiculobullous lesions, most commonly on the limbs, scalp and trunk. These lesions are replaced by linear verrucous plaques within days to weeks. Over time, the verrucous plaques disappear and streaks of reticulate hyperpigmentation develop, which can last until adulthood.

v. Other associated findings seen in IP include missing and conical teeth, linear absence of hair and sweat glands, dystrophic nails, ocular anomalies such as strabismus and cataracts, neurologic abnormalities such as seizures or developmental delay and skeletal defects such as skull anomalies or scoliosis.

vi. In the initial diagnosis and work-up of IP, a multidisciplinary approach is recommended, including general pediatrics, medical genetics, ophthalmology and dermatology. Other potential subspecialties that may be involved include neurology for neurologic abnormalities and orthopedics for skeletal defects.

CASE 88

X-linked ichthyosis

QUESTION 88

An 8-month-old infant presents to the pediatric dermatology clinic with his mother for the evaluation of dry scaly skin that has been unresponsive to topical emollients. The patient's mother states that he has had dry scaly skin for most of his life, but it has never been as severe as this. She also notes a birthing history of prolonged labor, resulting in cesarean section. Otherwise, the patient's past medical history since birth has been unremarkable and he has reached all appropriate developmental milestones. On examination, there are dark brown adherent scales on the extremities, trunk and neck with sparing of the face, palms, soles and skinfolds (88).

88

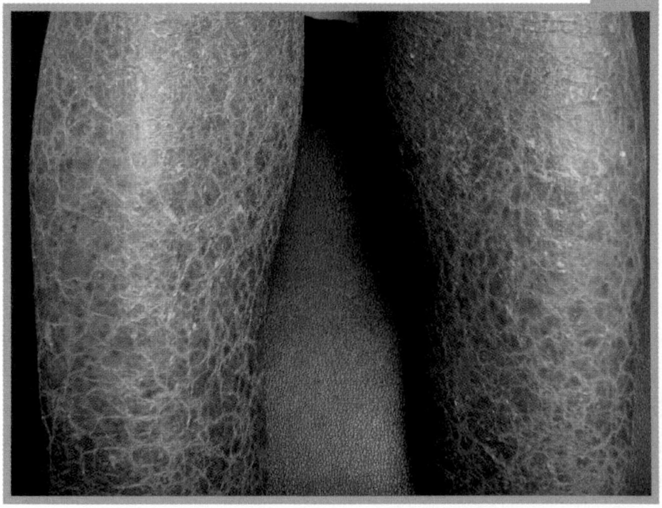

i. What is the deficiency and pathogenesis of this disease?

ii. How is the patient's birth history related to this disease?

iii. What other conditions should the patient's pediatrician screen for?

iv. How is this condition treated?

Answer 88

i. This patient presents with steroid sulfatase deficiency, also known as X-linked recessive ichthyosis. Along with ichthyosis vulgaris, steroid sulfatase deficiency is one of the more common ichthyoses with an estimated incidence of 1 in 2000 to 9500 male births. Seen almost exclusively in males, it is caused by a deletion or inactivating mutation of the entire *STS* gene on chromosome X, leading to the absence of or marked decrease in steroid sulfatase activity and subsequent inability to hydrolyze cholesterol sulfate and dehydroepiandrosterone sulfate (DHEAS). Impaired hydrolysis leads to accumulation of cholesterol 3-sulfate in the epidermis, which inhibits transglutaminase-1, leading to abnormal cornification and clinical scaling of the skin.

In the neonatal period, steroid sulfatase deficiency may present with mild erythroderma followed by peeling of large translucent scales. As infants grow older, they develop darker brown or characteristically 'dirty' appearing polygonal scales that almost always involve the neck and often involve the trunk and extremities. Flexural areas are often spared. Unlike ichthyosis vulgaris, this condition does not typically improve with age.

ii. Prolonged labor or failure to initiate labor can be seen in women with an affected fetus. Steroid sulfatase deficiency in the placenta can cause low or absent levels of estrogen in the urine and amniotic fluid, which causes insufficient dilation of the cervix, often requiring cesarean section for delivery.

iii. Patients with steroid sulfatase deficiency have a 20-fold increased incidence of cryptorchidism and have a higher risk for developing testicular cancer and hypogonadism. Asymptomatic corneal opacities can be seen in up to 50% of patients, and other rare associated non-cutaneous findings include seizures, developmental delay and acute lymphoblastic leukemia.

iv. Treatment involves the application of topical humectants, keratolytics and retinoids. Systemic treatment is rarely indicated.

CASE 89

Lamellar ichthyosis

QUESTION 89

A 23-year-old woman presents for the evaluation of dry, scaly skin. She reports a history of extremely dry and scaly skin throughout her life, from birth. She has tried numerous topical emollients and keratolytics with only mild–moderate improvement. She reports a family history of dry, scaly skin, but does not think any family member has had cutaneous disease as severe as hers. On examination, there are large plate-like scales on the trunk and extremities that are centrally attached with raised borders, with some areas showing superficial fissures (89a, b).

89a

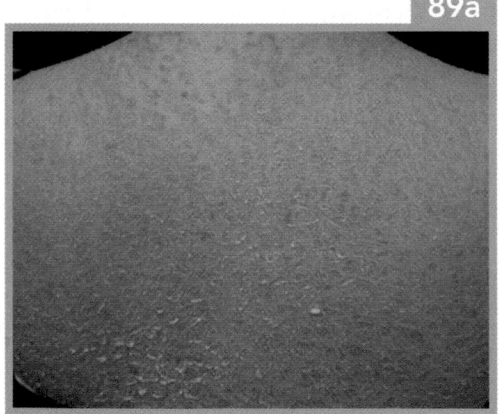

89b

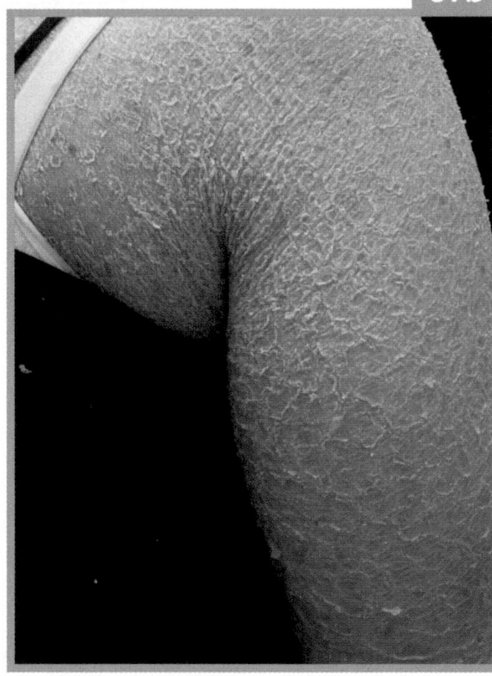

i. What is the diagnosis and genetic defect?

ii. How does this condition present at birth, and what are the potential complications?

iii. What treatments are available?

Answer 89

i. The patient presents with lamellar ichthyosis, an autosomal recessive congenital ichthyosis. The most common mutation observed in patients with classic lamellar ichthyosis is in the gene *TGM1*, which leads to transglutaminase-1 deficiency. This deficiency leads to disturbances in the process of cornification and desquamation of the normal epidermis. It is seen most often in patients of Northern European descent or in populations with consanguinity. Lamellar ichthyosis can also be seen less commonly in patients of Northern African descent, which is associated with the presence of a mutation in *ABCA12*, which is responsible for transporting lipid substrates across cell membranes.

ii. Neonates with classic lamellar ichthyosis present at birth with a collodion membrane, which is a taut transparent membrane resembling plastic wrap encasing the body, composed of thickened stratum corneum. After birth, the membrane becomes dry and is replaced by large scales that are brown, plate-like and form a mosaic pattern. Potential complications of lamellar ichthyosis are ectropion, eclabium or hypoplasia of the nasal cartilage.

iii. The mainstay of treatment is the use of emollients and humectants to reduce the amount of scaling. The use of topical products containing keratolytics such as α-hydroxy, lactic and salicylic acids can be used. Topical retinoids can also be helpful but may cause irritation to the skin. Severe forms of this disease can be treated with oral retinoids such as isotretinoin and acitretin.

CASE 90

Nevoid basal cell carcinoma syndrome

QUESTION 90

An 8-year-old Hispanic girl was referred to dermatology after she presented to a dentist with a complaint of tooth and jaw pain. On panoramic X-ray, there were three keratocystic odontogenic tumours, which were subsequently removed surgically, with histology confirming the diagnosis. She currently lives with her father, who reports that her mother had similar issues requiring repeated surgeries. Physical examination was notable for greater than three palmar pits on her bilateral hands and feet (90a, b).

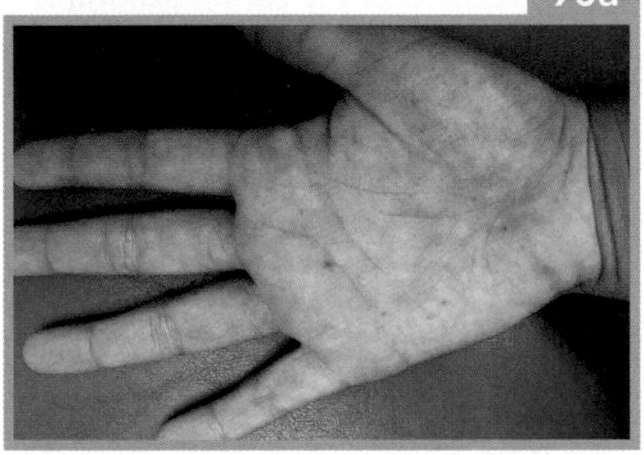
90a

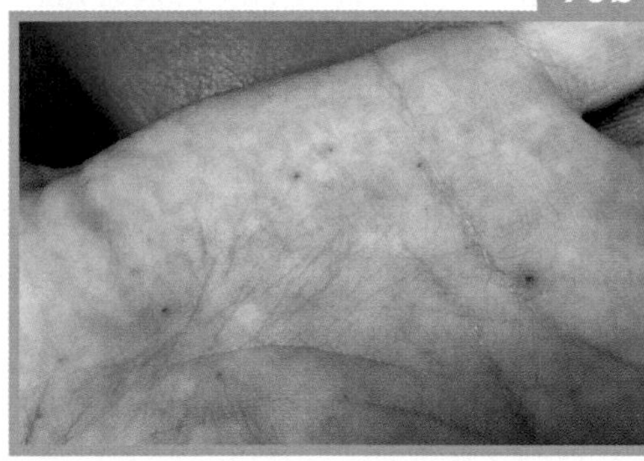
90b

i. What is the gene mutation seen in this disorder?

ii. What are the characteristic findings seen on chest X-ray and head imaging?

iii. What neoplasms are patients with this genetic syndrome at risk for?

Answer 90

i. This patient presents with a constellation of findings consistent with nevoid basal cell carcinoma (NBCC) syndrome, also known as Gorlin syndrome. This rare, autosomal dominant condition is caused by a mutation in the *PTCH1* gene, located in chromosome 9. The *PTCH1* gene is a tumour suppressor gene that encodes the sonic hedgehog transmembrane receptor protein that interacts with signalling proteins that play an important role in controlling cell proliferation.

ii. NBCC syndrome manifests in multiple organ systems. In the skin, it often presents with multiple basal cell carcinomas or a basal cell carcinoma at an early age. In addition, palmoplantar pits, milium and epidermoid cysts are commonly seen. Other manifestations include odontogenic keratocysts of the jaw, which can be painful and have malignant potential, as well as skeletal anomalies in the ribs, bilamellar calcification of the falx cerebri, agenesis of the corpus callosum, congenital blindness and less commonly, mental retardation. On chest X-ray, skeletal anomalies of the ribs can be seen, such as bifid, fused or markedly splayed ribs. Imaging of the head can demonstrate calcification of the falx cerebri.

iii. Patients with NBCC syndrome are also at risk of developing other neoplasms, including medulloblastomas (usually during childhood), meningiomas, bilateral ovarian fibromas and cardiac fibromas.

The diagnosis of NBCC syndrome requires the presence of two major criteria or one major and two minor criteria, which are listed below.

Major criteria	Minor criteria
• Multiple BCCs at any age or one BCC before the age of 20 years • Odontogenic keratocysts of the jaw • ≥3 palmar or plantar pits • Calcification of the falx cerebri • Bifid, fused or splayed rubs • A first-degree relative with NBCC syndrome	• Macrocephaly • Congenital malformations, such as cleft lip/palate, frontal bossing, coarse facies, hypertelorism • Other skeletal deformities, such as syndactyly, pectus deformity • Radiographic abnormalities, such as bridging of the sella turcica • Vertebral anomalies, such as hemivertebrae, fusion or elongation of the vertebral bodies • Bilateral ovarian fibromas • Medulloblastoma

CASE 91

Tuberous sclerosis

QUESTION 91

A 10-year-old girl was seen in the dermatology clinic for mild acne. Her parents tried over-the-counter 2% salicylic acid wash and 5% benzoyl peroxide wash without success before starting adapalene 0.1% cream. At her last well-child examination, she was referred to dermatology for further evaluation due to lack of response to therapy. Her past medical history is notable for cardiac rhabdomyomas, renal cysts and infantile seizures. On examination, there were numerous small reddish papules along the malar cheeks, nose and chin (91a). There were also several large hypopigmented patches on the trunk and extremities, and a cluster of soft, fleshy papules on the lower central back (91b).

91a

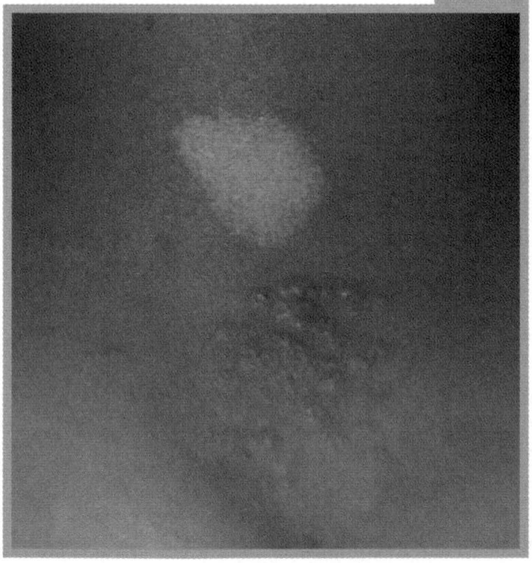

91b

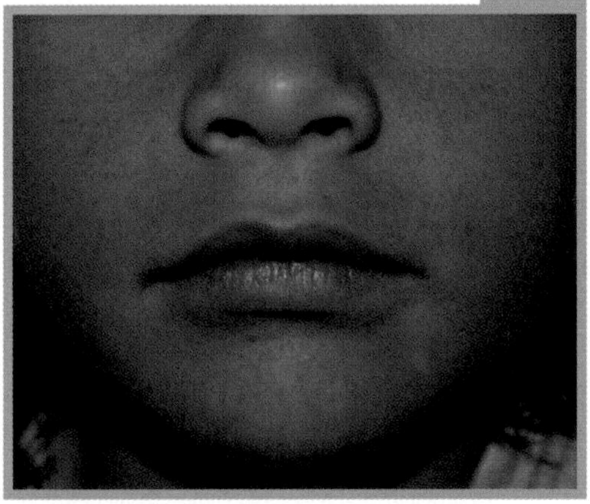

i. What is the most common mutation seen in this diagnosis?

ii. What are the major and minor criteria for diagnosis?

iii. What screening tests are recommended after the diagnosis?

iv. What findings are seen in the lungs of some of these patients, most commonly women of childbearing potential?

Answer 91

i. This patient has tuberous sclerosis complex (TSC), a neurocutaneous disease that is inherited in an autosomal dominant fashion or due to spontaneous mutations in up to 75% of the cases. The most common mutation seen in TSC is in the *TSC2* gene on chromosome 16, which encodes a protein called tuberin. A less common mutation is seen in the *TSC1* gene on chromosome 9, which encodes hamartin. A mutation in *TSC2* is seen more often than in *TSC1*, in an approximately 3:1 ratio, and is also associated with a more severe phenotype.

Clinically, TSC is characterized by cutaneous findings, such as facial angiofibromas, hypomelanotic macules, shagreen patches, periungual fibromas and café-au-lait macules. Additional clinical findings include retinal hamartomas, achromatic retinal patches, pitted enamel of the teeth, gingival fibromas, multiple bilateral renal angiomyoplipomas, renal cysts and/or renal carcinomas, seizures, subependymal nodules and cortical tubers, infantile spasms, mental retardation and myocardial rhabdomyomas.

ii. There are 11 major and 9 minor criteria for the diagnosis of TSC. A diagnosis of definite TSC can be made by the presence of either two major features or one major plus two minor features. The diagnosis of TSC is considered probable in the setting of one major plus one minor feature and possible in the presence of either one major or two or more minor features. They are as follows:

Major criteria	Minor criteria
• Facial angiofibromas or forehead plaque • Non-traumatic ungual or periungual fibromas • Hypomelanotic macules (≥3) • Shagreen patch (connective tissue nevus) • Multiple retinal nodular hamartomas • Cortical tubers • Subependymal nodules • Subependymal giant cell astrocytoma • Renal angiomyoplipoma • Cardiac rhabdomyoma (single or multiple) • Lymphangioleiomyomatosis	• 'Confetti' hypopigmented skin lesions • Multiple dental enamel pits • Gingival fibromas • Retinal achromic patch • Cerebral white matter radial migration lines • Multiple renal cysts • Hamartomatous rectal polyps • Bone cysts • Non-renal hamartoma

iii. As TSC can potentially affect nearly every organ system, a multidisciplinary approach is necessary for the management of TSC. After the diagnosis of TSC, comprehensive developmental assessments at school may be required to monitor educational or behavioural concerns. Screening for ophthalmologic involvement should be performed as needed, as well as screening cranial computed tomographies (CTs) or magnetic resonance imagings (MRIs) every 1–3 years and a renal ultrasound every 1–3 years (or more frequently in the setting of known renal lesions).

iv. Lymphangioleiomyomatosis, which was historically thought to be a rare clinical finding in TSC, is seen in up to one-third of women with TSC. It is characterized by the presence of cystic lesions on CT imaging, and estrogen is thought to play a role in the development of this manifestation of TSC, as it is rarely seen in men.

CASE 92

Hailey–Hailey disease

QUESTION 92

A 42-year-old woman presents to the dermatology clinic for the evaluation of a painful rash in her skinfolds. The rash has been present for about 1 year, but has progressively worsened and spread from involving the axillae to the groin folds and lower back. It is worse during the summer, especially with sweating and friction. She also notes malodorous drainage from these areas that require her to change her clothes twice a day. She has been evaluated by her primary care physician and treated with topical nystatin cream and powder for intertrigo, without improvement. On examination, there are arcuate and polycyclic well-demarcated plaques with central areas of erosion and an erythematous, scaly border (92a, b).

92a

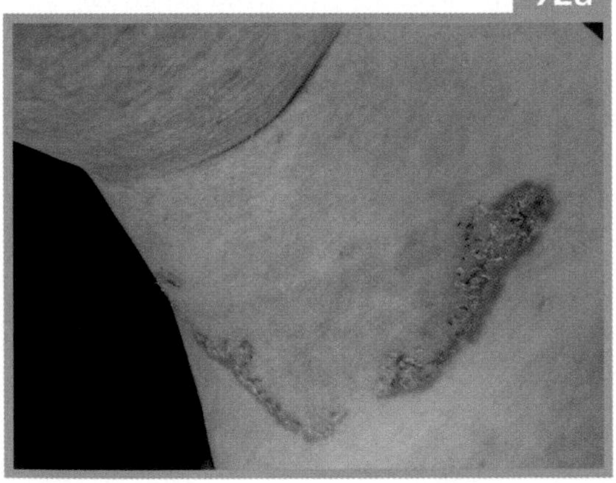

92b

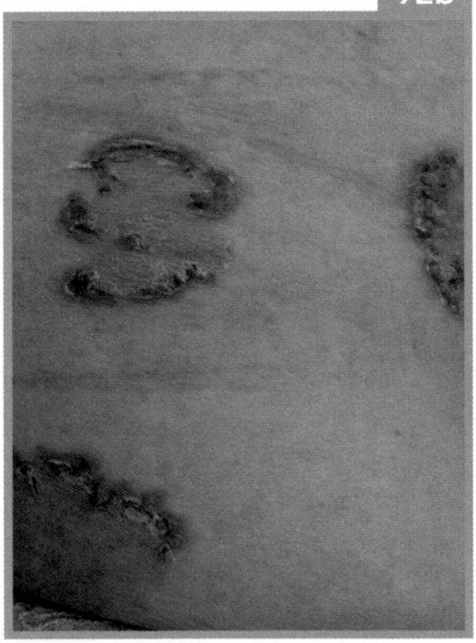

i. What is the diagnosis and aetiology of this condition?

ii. What are the characteristic histological findings?

iii. What treatments are available for this disease?

Answer 92

i. The patient presents with Hailey–Hailey disease, also known as familial benign chronic pemphigus. This is an autosomal dominant disease caused by a mutation in the *ATP2C1* gene. Hailey–Hailey disease usually presents in adulthood and is characterized by the formation of flaccid vesicles that evolve into erosions, distributed in the intertriginous areas such as the axillae, groin, perianal region and inframammary region in women. Lesions can become crusted and vegetative and develop painful fissures.

ii. Histologically, Hailey–Hailey disease demonstrates acantholysis in the epidermis, often referred to as a 'dilapidated brick wall' in appearance. Although some features may overlap with Darier disease, which is also characterized by acantholysis, the presence of necrotic keratinocytes is not a prominent feature in Hailey–Hailey disease as it is in Darier disease, and the discohesion within the epidermis is more widespread in Hailey–Hailey disease.

iii. Wearing light, loose-fitting clothes can decrease sweating and friction, both of which can exacerbate Hailey–Hailey disease. Topical antimicrobial agents and bleach baths are often recommended to prevent secondary bacterial infection of chronic lesions. For topical treatment, corticosteroids are used often, however, they should be used at the lowest concentration necessary to avoid potential side effects of topical corticosteroids within intertriginous areas. There are also reports of the successful treatment with injection of botulinum toxin. There is no systemic medication that has demonstrated efficacy in large studies to date. There are anecdotal reports on the use of immunomodulatory medications such as prednisone, methotrexate and cyclosporine for patients with severe and refractory Hailey–Hailey disease.

PHOTODERMATOLOGIC DISORDERS

CASE 93

Grover's disease

QUESTION 93

A 71-year-old man presents to the dermatology clinic with a sudden-onset pruritic eruption on the chest and back. The day prior to developing this rash, he was outside shovelling snow. No one he lives with has similar symptoms. On examination, he has numerous excoriated small pink to red papules, some with overlying hemorrhagic crusting. He also has numerous seborrheic keratoses of the neck (93). He has not tried any treatment thus far.

93

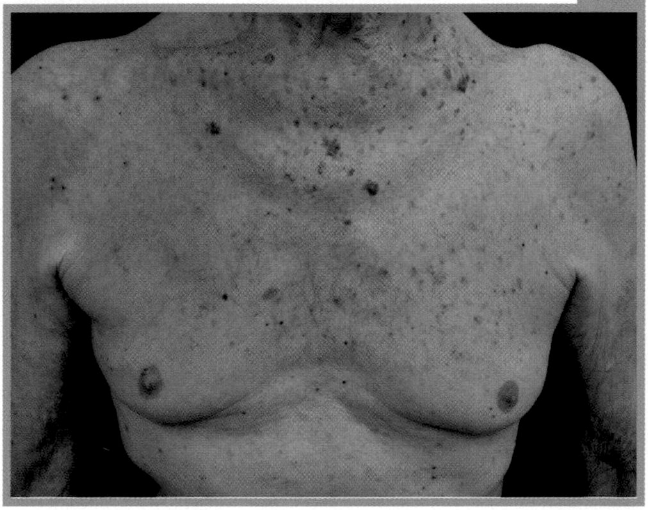

i. What is the diagnosis?

ii. What other conditions have similar findings histologically?

iii. What is the prognosis and available treatment options for this condition?

Answer 93

i. The patient presents with Grover's disease, also known as transient acantholytic dermatosis, which is characterized by an eruption of crusted, pruritic papules or vesicles that arise primarily on sun-exposed areas of the trunk. It is seen most often in middle-aged to elderly men with a history of significant photodamage. It is typically worse with sun exposure, sweating, and friction and patients will complain of flares during the summer season. The differential diagnosis includes folliculitis, miliaria rubra, chronic Darier disease, lichen planus-like keratoses and early pemphigus foliaceus.

ii. The characteristic histologic feature of Grover's disease is the presence of focal acantholysis or separation of the epidermal cells. Other conditions that can also demonstrate this feature prominently are Darier's disease and Hailey–Hailey disease. In contrast, although pemphigus vulgaris or pemphigus foliaceus will demonstrate acantholysis on histopathology, this is not seen in a focal pattern in these entities and can be easily distinguished.

iii. Grover's disease is a benign chronic condition, although it can be frustrating for many patients as therapy can be disappointing. Typical treatments include topical agents, such as corticosteroids, pramoxine and vitamin D analogues. Additional treatment with oral antihistamines can be used as adjunctive therapies.

CASE 94

Favre–Racouchot

QUESTION 94

A 67-year-old woman presents to the dermatology clinic for the evaluation of dark spots around her eyes. She states that she initially noticed a few spots, which developed over the past several years. She has tried to express the contents and notes a scant amount of black material. Her past medical history is notable for multiple nonmelanoma skin cancers of the scalp and face. On examination, there are multiple open comedones along the lateral and inferior aspects of the periorbital area, along with evidence of diffuse photodamage in the surrounding skin (94).

94

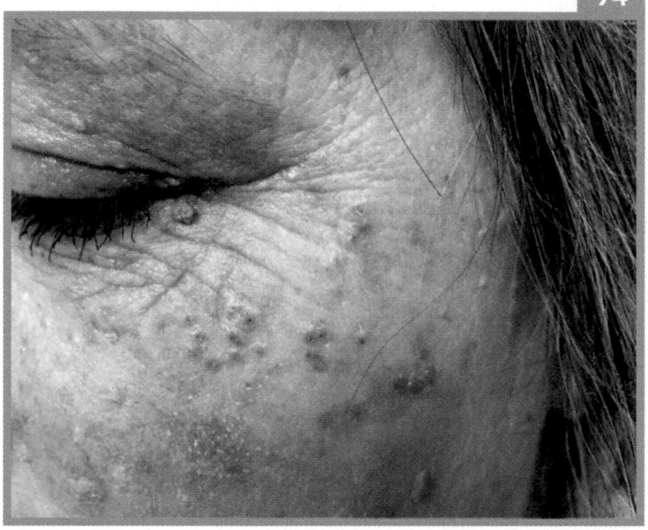

i. What is the diagnosis?

ii. What are the management options?

Answer 94

i. The lesions on this patient's face are characteristic of Favre–Racouchot syndrome, also known as solar comedones, which is the result of chronic sun exposure or photodamage to the skin. It is characterized by the development of large open or closed comedones on the lateral and inferior periorbital areas. These lesions are typically persistent and can recur.

Photoageing of the skin refers to the changes in the skin that occur due to long-term exposure to ultraviolet (UV) radiation. It is characterized by a chronic inflammatory response to UV light, with one of the prominent features being a loss of collagen fibres and actinic (solar) elastosis. The chronic inflammation caused by chronic UV exposure leads to the upregulation of proteases that degrade the extracellular matrix of the skin and the downregulation of collagen synthesis. UVA radiation, which spans wavelengths 315–400 nm, is thought to play a major role in photoageing due to its ability to penetrate deeper in the dermis.

ii. First-line therapy for Favre–Racouchot and other chronic sun-induced lesions is consistent sun protection. For Favre–Racouchot, using oil-free sunscreen and non-comedogenic facial products can be helpful. Topical retinoids can help decrease the appearance of the affected areas and also improve the overall complexion of photodamaged skin. Open comedones can be extracted but often recur and require repeated treatments.

SKIN FINDINGS FROM EXTERNAL OR PHYSICAL AGENTS

CASE 95

Chondrodermatitis nodularis helicis

QUESTION 95

A 75-year-old Caucasian woman with a history of osteoarthritis presents to the clinic with a 3-month history of an exquisitely painful, non-healing nodule on the right antihelix, which prevents her from sleeping on her right side. She has tried warm compresses and antibacterial ointment but has not had any relief from her symptoms. On examination, there is an erythematous papule with central ulceration on the right mid-helix of the ear (95).

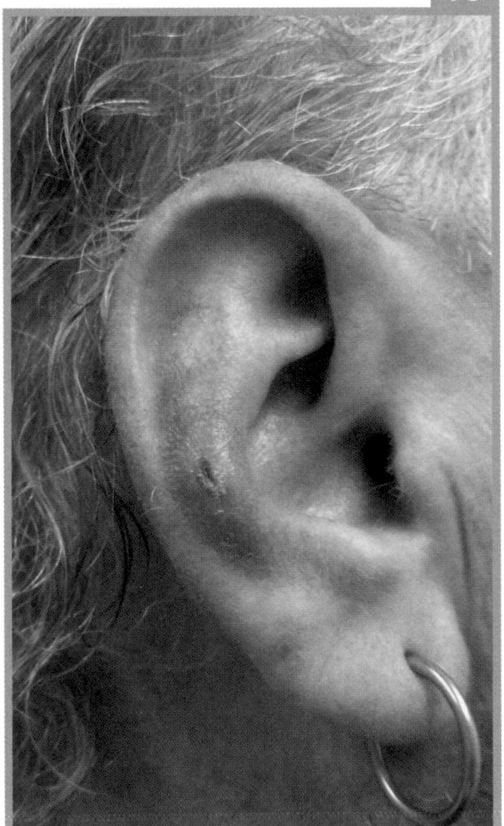
95

i. What is the diagnosis?

ii. What are the treatment options for this skin lesion?

Answer 95

i. The patient has an exquisitely painful lesion on the ear that is characteristic of chondrodermatitis nodularis chronica helicis (CNH). CNH can present with varying degrees of erythema, ulceration or a central crater, with or without crust. CNH is predominantly seen in men, with an estimated ratio of 10:1. However, in women, antihelix lesions are more common. CNH lesions often resemble cutaneous carcinomas, due to their appearance and location on the ear, and can be distinguished by histologic findings. Histologically, there is characteristic epidermal hyperplasia and hyperkeratosis with increased vascularity and degenerative changes in the cartilage.

ii. There are numerous therapies that have been described in the literature for CNH, with varying reports of efficacy and few controlled studies. Surgical modalities include wedge resection, punch and graft technique and simple excision. Other destructive measures such as electrodessication and curettage and cryotherapy have been reported. Other treatment options include topical and intralesional corticosteroids, injectable collagen, carbon dioxide laser and topical nitroglycerin. Supportive, non-invasive therapies include the use of a doughnut pillow or moulded prosthesis which alleviates the symptoms of pain.

CASE 96

Coma bullae

QUESTION 96

A 27-year-old man presents to the emergency room after being found unconscious and unresponsive. Cardiopulmonary resuscitation was initiated by first responders and the patient was intubated, found to have opioid overdose and alcohol intoxication and admitted to the intensive care unit for further treatment. On his third day of hospitalization, the medical team consulted the inpatient dermatologist after noticing the formation of blisters on the palmar eminence and volar wrist. On examination, there were tense, fluid-filled bullae with surrounding erythema and induration on the palm and volar wrist (96).

96

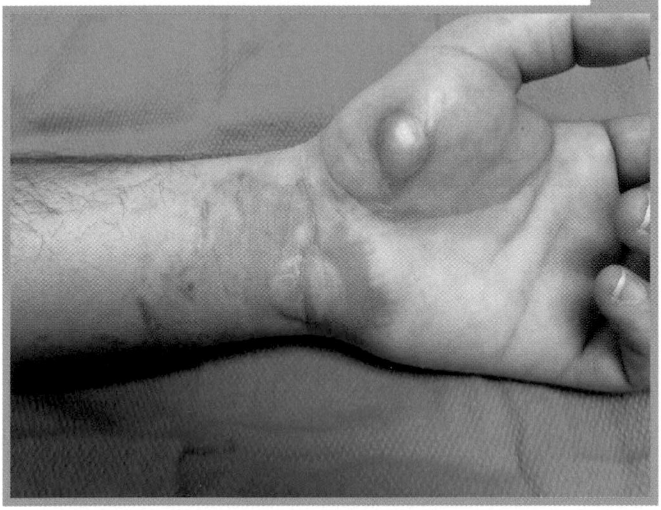

i. What is the most likely diagnosis?

ii. What are the characteristic features of this disease on histopathological examination?

iii. What is the treatment of choice for this disease?

Answer 96

i. This patient developed coma blisters or coma bullae, which are blisters that develop at sites of maximal pressure in patients with a history of loss of consciousness, neurologic diseases or prolonged immobilization. They typically begin as a blanchable patch or plaque within the first 24 hours and progress to blisters or erosions with 48–72 hours after the onset of coma. Although the first reports of coma blisters were observed in association with barbiturate overdose patients, other causes of coma including other overdoses such as opioids, carbon monoxide poisoning, viral encephalitis, metabolic encephalopathies, head trauma or cerebrovascular accidents (CVAs) have been described in association with coma bullae. Although the true pathogenesis of coma bullae is not well understood, pressure, friction and local hypoxia are thought to be contributing factors.

ii. The blisters are mostly subepidermal, but intraepidermal blisters can be seen in the process of re-epithelialization of older lesions. A characteristic finding histologically is sweat gland necrosis and focal necrosis of the epithelium of the pilosebaceous follicles.

iii. Erosions heal spontaneously over 1–2 weeks, though residual scarring can occur in some patients. Frequent postural changes help resolve and prevent coma bullae.

CASE 97

Erythema ab igne

QUESTION 97

A 37-year-old woman presents with skin colour changes on the left lower leg. She states that she sustained a twisting injury to the left ankle about 1 year ago and still has pain, which she treats with ibuprofen and heat packs. No previous treatments have been attempted. She denies any pruritus or pain. On examination, there is an area of reticular hyperpigmentation overlying the dorsal ankle (97).

97

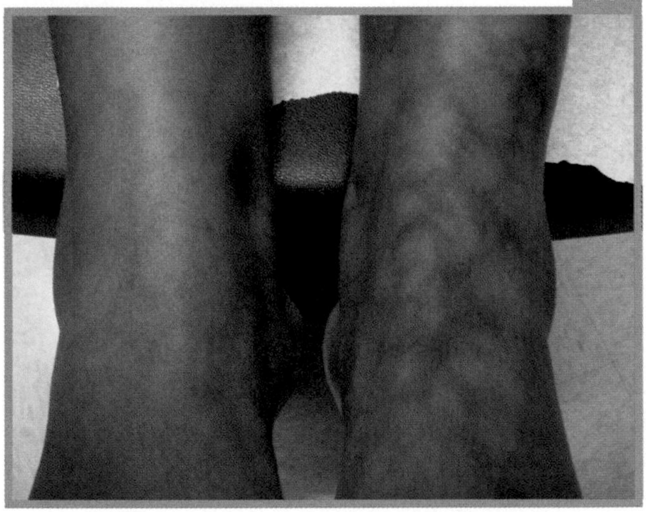

i. What is the most likely diagnosis, and what is the pathogenesis?

ii. What histologic findings are seen on skin biopsy?

iii. What additional concerns are associated with this condition?

Answer 97

i. This patient's history and clinical findings are consistent with erythema ab igne, also referred to as fire stains or toasted skin syndrome. It is characterized by localized areas of reticulated erythema and hyperpigmentation due to chronic exposure to heat below the threshold of a thermal burn. Initially, the macular colour changes are transient and easily blanchable. As heat exposure continues over time, it leads to dusky hyperpigmentation that leads to fixed colour changes that are no longer blanchable. Later lesions of erythema ab igne can demonstrate epidermal atrophy, appear keratotic or lead to bullae formation. Although, the exact pathophysiology is unknown, repeated exposure to heat below 45°C (113°F) results in a reticulated erythema in a pattern that corresponds with the dermal venous plexus. Common heat sources reported to cause erythema ab igne include heating pads, hot water bottles, heating blankets, heated car seats, heated reclining chairs and laptops/computers (often affecting the anterior thighs). Additional causes include open fires, coal stoves, steam radiators and electric stoves/heaters.

ii. On skin biopsy, early histopathologic changes are epidermal atrophy, vasodilation and dermal pigmentation with melanin and hemosiderin. Later lesions of erythema ab igne demonstrate more prominent epidermal atrophy with flattening of the rete ridges. Focal hyperkeratosis and dyskeratosis with squamous atypia can be seen. Lesions in the legs demonstrate more prominent hemosiderin deposition and prominent telangiectasias.

iii. Due to the presence of epidermal atypia, which is comparable to that of actinic keratoses, the possible development of cutaneous squamous cell carcinoma or Merkel cell carcinoma is a major long-term concern associated with erythema ab igne. There are anecdotal reports of treating the area with topical 5-fluorouracil.

CASE 98

Keloid

QUESTION 98

A 46-year-old Hispanic man presents to the clinic for the evaluation of a large scar on his chest. He does not remember any preceding injury or trauma to this area, and the area of scar involvement has increased over a course of months. He has associated itching, tenderness and sensitivity in the area. On examination, there is a large pink firm plaque on the central chest (98).

98

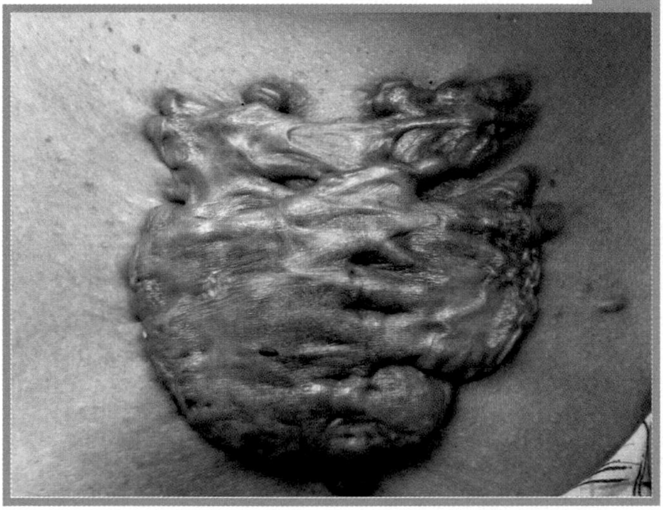

i. What is the diagnosis?

ii. What systemic diseases can this diagnosis be associated with?

iii. What is the prognosis?

Answer 98

i. This patient presents with a keloid, a sign of abnormal wound healing. In comparison to a hypertrophic scar, another form of abnormal wound healing confined to an area of prior insult, keloids extend beyond the wound margin or occur spontaneously in individuals without any inciting injury at all. Both hypertrophic scars and keloids form as a result of local fibroblast proliferation and excessive collagen production. In keloids, collagen synthesis is approximately 20-fold greater than in normal non-injured skin.

Keloids differ from normal and hypertrophic scars in that they do not have to be preceded by injury, and the onset of a keloid is often delayed, up to several months. It is usually associated with pruritus, pain with erythema, and/or pigmentary changes. As keloids extend beyond the original wound margin, it extends with claw-like extensions.

Histologically, keloids are characterized by the presence of haphazard, thick, hyalinized, homogenous collagen bundles with mucinous ground substance and an increased number of fibroblasts.

ii. Epidemiologically, keloids are a sporadic finding seen more commonly in black and Hispanic populations, often with a familial tendency. Keloids can also be seen in keloidal forms of scleroderma, morphea, type IV Ehlers–Danlos syndrome, carcinoma en cuirasse or in rare inherited conditions including Rubinstein–Taybi and Goeminne syndromes.

iii. The prognosis of keloids is poor. Lesions rarely regress spontaneously and are often resistant to treatment. Keloids are best treated with a combination of methods including surgery, radiation therapy, intralesional injections with corticosteroids (10–40 mg/mL), verapamil or 5-fluorouracil. Topical treatments such as imiquimod, tacrolimus and retinoids have been reported.

CASE 99

Aquagenic wrinkling of the palms

QUESTION 99

A 19-year-old college student with a history of asthma presents with painful thickening and textural changes in the skin on her palms. She has recently started working at a coffee shop in the evenings and believes that her symptoms are most prominent when she washes dishes. She has tried using emollients but the symptoms persist. After emersion in water for 1 minute, there is palmar wrinkling and white-appearing papular changes in the skin of the palms (99).

99

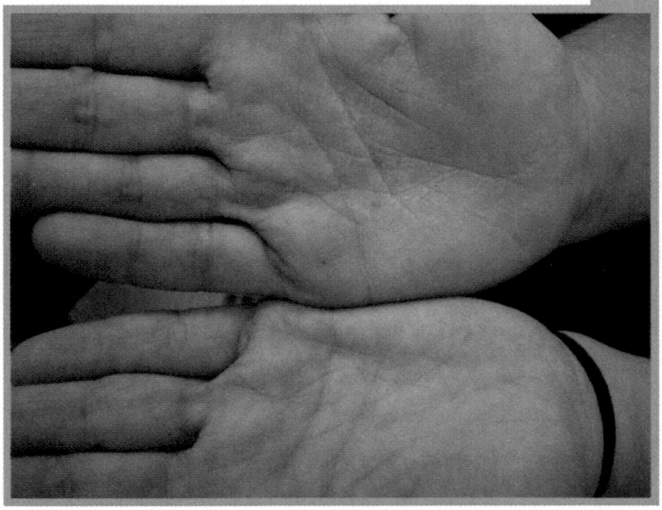

i. What is the diagnosis?

ii. What genetic disease is associated with this dermatologic condition?

Answer 99

i. The patient presents with aquagenic palmoplantar keratoderma or aquagenic wrinkling of the palms (AWP). This condition is characterized by transient thickening and white or translucent 'pebbly' changes in the palms or soles after immersion in water. Patients may also experience pain, edema, burning and a tingling sensation. Seen more commonly in women, the typical time of onset is in the second decade of life.

ii. Aquagenic wrinkling of the palms is associated with the F508 cystic fibrosis transmembrane conductance regular gene mutation and is highly prevalent among patients with cystic fibrosis (CF). Studies have documented a prevalence of AWP in up to 84% of patients with CF. AWP in a young person deserves further consideration, including a complete review of systems with a particular emphasis on the history of sinus disease, nasal polyps, wheezing or reactive airway disease. AWP can also be seen in normal individuals. In normal control groups, palmar wrinkling can be observed in individuals after approximately 12 minutes of water submersion. In contrast, patients with CF with AWP develop palmar changes within 2 minutes and CF carriers with AWP develop changes within 7 minutes.

CASE 100

Granulomatous tattoo reaction

QUESTION 100

A 36-year-old woman presents to the dermatology clinic for the evaluation of a raised pink plaque within a tattoo. She got the tattoo inked approximately 6 months ago without any adverse effect until 3 weeks before her visit to the clinic. She initially noticed an elevated area within the tattoo that subsequently enlarged and became scaly and pruritic. She has other tattoos on other areas of her body that are not affected. On physical examination, there are erythematous scaly plaques within the ink margins of specific areas of her tattoo with overlying crust and some areas of erosion (100).

100

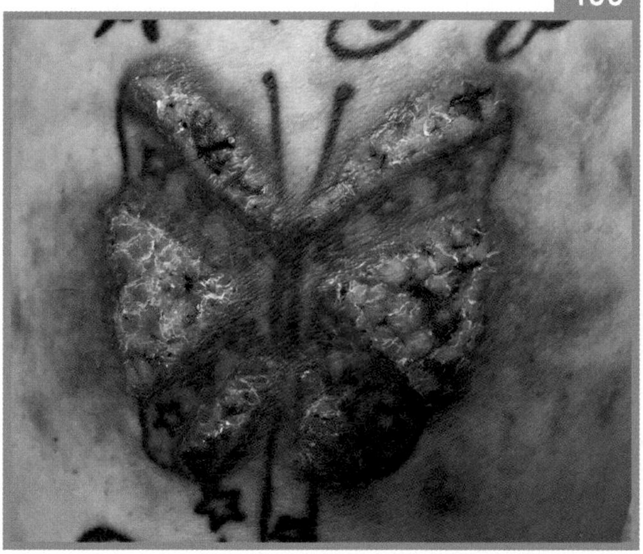

i. What tattoo colour is most commonly associated with this reaction?

ii. What chemicals are used to make this colour?

iii. What are some of the available treatment options?

Answer 100

i. The patient presents with a granulomatous reaction to a tattoo, which is seen most commonly as a reaction to red tattoo ink. As seen in this patient's clinical image, a granulomatous reaction can be seen within the areas where red tattoo dye was deposited in the skin, while the other areas of the tattoo are uninvolved.

Granulomatous tattoo reactions are characterized by erythematous nodules or plaques with lichenoid or eczematous features. Based on the extent of inflammation, there can be associated tenderness and erythema.

ii. Red tattoo pigment is composed of mercury sulfide or cinnabar, ferric hydrate, sandalwood or brazilwood.

iii. There is a wide variety of options for the treatment of granulomatous tattoo reactions. Tattoo removal can be performed with different lasers, such as Q-switched ruby, alexandrite and Nd:YAG, although this may lead to scarring. Lasers should not be used to treat patients with inflamed tattoos, as there is a risk of inducing a systemic reaction. For patients who are not able to undergo laser tattoo removal, topical or intralesional corticosteroids can lead to symptom relief.

INDEX